WHAT WORRIES WOMEN MOST

Your Medical Questions Answered

Dedication

To every woman who worries about her health.

With special thanks to my mother Nina, and my granny, Joan, who coped with all my worries when I was growing up. And to Richard who copes with them now.

Author and Publisher's Note

A book such as this can only give general assistance. Each patient's symptoms and conditions vary. If you have any medical problems that worry you, you should seek professional advice from your usual medical practitioner without delay.

WHAT WORRIES WOMEN MOST

Your Medical Questions Answered

Dr Sarah Brewer

Piccadilly Press · London

Copyright © Sarah Brewer, 1993

All rights reserved. No part of this publication may be reproduced, stored in a retrieval system, or transmitted, in any form or by any means electronic, mechanical, photocopying, recording or otherwise, without the prior permission of the copyright owner.

The right of Sarah Brewer to be identified as Author of this work has been asserted by her in accordance with the Copyright, Designs and Patents Act 1988.

Phototypeset by Goodfellow & Egan, Cambridge
Printed and bound by WBC, Bridgend, Glamorgan
for the publishers, Piccadilly Press Ltd,
5 Castle Road, London NW1 8PR

A catalogue record for this book is available from the British Library

ISBN 1-85340-215-X

Dr Sarah Brewer divides her time between central London and Devon. After qualifying at Cambridge, she practised as a GP for many years. She is now a medical editor although she continues to work part-time as a doctor. She writes regularly for *Woman's Weekly*, the *Northern Sunday News & Echo*, the *Birmingham Evening Mail* and *Here's Health*. She has collaborated on one book, *The Bluffer's Guide to Sex*. This is her second one, and her first for Piccadilly Press.

INTRODUCTION

If you worry about your health, or are just interested in the facts and statistics that make medicine so vitally interesting, read this book. It will put your mind to rest – or galvanise you into seeking immediate necessary treatment.

Family doctors are currently under a great deal of pressure. Patients realise this and, at the expense of their own health, continue to let problems fester.

As a GP, I worry about the potentially serious problems of patients who are unable to pluck up the courage to talk to their physician. Having written *Dear Doctor* columns for newspapers and magazines, I am constantly concerned by the number of serious conditions patients seek advice about through the popular press.

WHAT WORRIES WOMEN MOST covers the vast majority of queries received in my mail bag each week. If a particular condition hasn't been addressed which distresses you, write and tell us and we will include it in future editions. In the meantime, however, do seek the help of your GP. A large part of our job is concerned with reassuring or advising on non-serious worries as well as potentially serious conditions.

CONTENTS

SEX 15–31

1. Can a man tell if a woman's a virgin? 15
2. Can a man tell if I fake an orgasm? 16
3. What should I know about orgasms? 17
4. What is a 'normal' sex drive? 18
5. Am I frigid? 19
6. What is the G-spot? 20
7. Is oral sex safe? 21
8. Is anal sex normal? 22
9. Is masturbation harmful? 23
10. What happens to sperm inside me? 23
11. What are the symptoms and signs of sexually transmitted diseases? 24
12. How common are HIV and Aids? 25
13. Can heterosexual sex pass on HIV? 27
14. What is safer sex? 28
15. What are pheromones? 29
16. Why does sex sometimes hurt? 30

CONTRACEPTION AND ABORTION 32–45

17. How does the combined pill work? 33
18. How does the mini-pill work? 35
19. What should I do if I forget to take a combined pill? 36
20. What should I do if I forget to take a mini-pill? 37

WHAT WORRIES WOMEN MOST

21.	How long after unprotected sex does the morning-after pill work?	37
22.	What other methods of emergency contraception are available?	38
23.	Is inserting a diaphragm easy?	39
24.	How does the contraceptive injection work?	41
25.	Is sterilisation really irreversible?	42
26.	Can you get pregnant during a period?	42
27.	What new forms of contraception are being developed?	42
28.	What are the legal requirements for termination of pregnancy?	43
29.	What happens during termination of pregnancy?	44

PERIODS 46–54

30.	What is a normal menstrual cycle?	46
31.	Why are my periods heavy?	49
32.	Why are my periods painful?	50
33.	Why are my periods irregular?	51
34.	What will my doctor do if I consult her/him about my periods?	52
35.	What is Toxic Shock Syndrome?	53

PRE-MENSTRUAL SYNDROME 55–58

36.	What are the symptoms of PMS and what causes them?	56
37.	What treatments are available for PMS?	57

Contents

INFERTILITY 59–66

38.	Why can't I get pregnant?	60
39.	How are grandmothers able to conceive?	62
40.	What tests are done for infertility?	63
41.	What methods are available to help me achieve pregnancy?	64

PREGNANCY 67–78

42.	Is pre-conception preparation important?	68
43.	How can I tell if I'm pregnant?	70
44.	Why does miscarriage occur?	71
45.	What tests can ensure that my baby is normal?	72
46.	Is it safe to take exercise during pregnancy?	74
47.	What methods of pain relief are available during labour? Are they safe?	74
48.	Will I need an episiotomy?	76
49.	Is breast milk better than the bottle?	77

CYSTITIS 79–81

50.	Why do I keep getting cystitis?	79
51.	What self-help remedies are available for cystitis?	80

STRESS INCONTINENCE 82–84

52.	What causes stress incontinence?	82
53.	What can be done for stress incontinence?	83

WHAT WORRIES WOMEN MOST

THRUSH 85–87

54. What are the symptoms of genital thrush? 85
55. Why do I get recurrent thrush? 85
56. What thrush treatments are available? 86

VAGINAL DISCHARGE 88–92

57. What causes excess vaginal discharge? 89
58. Why do vaginal discharges smell? 90

HYSTERECTOMY/PROBLEMS THAT CAN LEAD TO HYSTERECTOMY 93–101

59. Do I need a hysterectomy? 93
60. What are fibroids? 94
61. What is a prolapse? 95
62. What is endometriosis? 96
63. What is pelvic inflammatory disease? 96
64. What happens during hysterectomy? 98
65. Will I lose my ovaries when having a hysterectomy? 99
66. Will I be less feminine or lose my sex drive after a hysterectomy? 99
67. What are the alternatives to hysterectomy? 100

MENOPAUSE 102–117

68. Will my sex drive dwindle after the menopause? 103
69. What are the risks and benefits of hormone replacement therapy? 104
70. Can I have the HRT patch? 108

CONTENTS

71. *Will HRT mean my periods return?*   108
72. *What is the significance of post-menopausal bleeding?*   109
73. *When is it safe to stop using contraception after the menopause?*   110
74. *What alternatives to HRT are available for treating menopausal symptoms?*   112
75. *Why do women get osteoporosis?*   113
76. *Can osteoporosis be prevented?*   114
77. *Who should have bone density screening?*   115

BREAST CANCER   118–123

78. *How should I check my breasts for lumps?*   118
79. *What should I do if I find a breast lump?*   120
80. *What is a mammogram and who should have one?*   121
81. *What causes breast pain?*   122

COSMETIC BREAST SURGERY   124–128

82. *Can breasts easily be made larger or smaller?*   124
83. *Do breast implants cause cancer?*   125
84. *Do breast implants cause auto-immune disease or other problems?*   126

THE AGEING SKIN   129–137

85. *Why do I get wrinkles?*   130
86. *What are collagen injections?*   130
87. *Does the anti-wrinkle treatment tretinoin really work?*   132
88. *What happens during a face-lift?*   133

WHAT WORRIES WOMEN MOST

89. What causes stretch marks?   134
90. What can be done about excess body hair?   135

ACNE   138–140

91. Why do I get spots?   138
92. What treatments are available for acne?   139

HEALTHY DIET   141–147

93. What is cholesterol and what is a safe blood level?   142
94. How much fat should my diet contain?   144
95. Is the Mediterranean diet really good for the heart?   146

SLIMMING   148–158

96. What is my 'ideal' weight?   148
97. How many calories do I need?   149
98. Why am I fat? Is it my hormones or my metabolism?   151
99. What is the best way to lose weight?   152
100. Are slimming pills safe?   153
101. Are Very Low Calorie diets safe?   154
102. What causes bulimia or anorexia nervosa?   155
103. Should I take vitamin pills?   156
104. How much exercise do I need?   157
105. What operations can help me lose weight?   157

ALCOHOL   159–162

106. How much can I safely drink?   159

Contents

107.	What effects does alcohol have on the body?	160
108.	What are the signs of alcohol dependency?	161

SMOKING 163–167

109.	Why is smoking unhealthy?	164
110.	What is the easiest way to stop smoking?	165

PSYCHIATRY 168–178

111.	What are the symptoms of stress?	168
112.	How can I lower my stress levels?	169
113.	What can be done about anxiety?	171
114.	What can be done about phobias?	173
115.	What causes post-natal depression?	174
116.	What are the symptoms of depressive illness?	176
117.	Are sleeping tablets harmful or addictive?	177

CANCER 179–187

118.	What are the commonest cancers?	180
119.	Are cancers hereditary or infectious?	181
120.	How is cancer treated?	182
121.	What happens during a cervical smear?	183
122.	Should I have a cervical smear?	184
123.	What does an abnormal smear signify?	185
124.	What happens during a colposcopy?	187

CELLULITE 188–189

125.	What is cellulite and how can it be minimised	188

SEX

Sex is an activity like eating, breathing and sleeping which is said to be totally instinctive. Despite this, we spend a lot of time worrying about doing it correctly.

'Proper' sex varies around the globe, with some practices so bizarre that if encountered in the western world a psychiatrist, strings of social workers and a grand jury would instantly be convened: penises are split in two (Aborigines) and implanted with opals and pearls (Thailand); labia are stitched together leaving a gap like a grain of rice (Sudan, Somalia) and clitorises are excised without the aid of anaesthesia (Middle East, Nigeria); children are taught foreplay and penetration by their parents (the Lepcha of the Himalayas) and some tribes (the Muria of India) expect daughters to lose their virginity by the age of six.

The more affluent a culture becomes, the more sex is thought of as recreational, but HIV and Aids have encouraged a widespread re-assessment of sexual values and promiscuity is now passé. Emphasis in the nineties is firmly on caring, quality, safety and love, which are all potent sources for worry.

1. Can a man tell if a woman's a virgin?

It's commonly believed that a woman is only a virgin if her hymen remains intact. This is incorrect. The hymen is merely a flap of skin which partially or completely occludes the vaginal entrance. Some females are born without one and in many cases, the

WHAT WORRIES WOMEN MOST

hymen is delicate enough to rupture undetected during activities such as bicycling. Occasionally, the hymen is more substantial and needs aggressive thrusting to break. This results in pain and bleeding – but the lack of these by no means indicates that a woman is not a virgin.

Tampons are often sufficient to break or stretch the hymen and permit the passage of a penis. Rarely, the hymen totally occludes the vagina so even menstrual flow is stemmed. This can result in litres of putrid blood accumulating in a condition known as haematocolpos.

Virginity is as much to do with state of mind as whether or not a woman has had penetrative sex. A confident virgin who has successfully used tampons, read all the textbooks and responds enthusiastically is unlikely to be identified as sexually naive. Most males couldn't care less whether a woman is a virgin. Over 30% actively prefer their partner to be experienced.

2. *Can a man tell if I fake an orgasm?*

If you do it well, no. A woman who has experienced orgasm through intercourse or masturbation will know her usual response. Some remain totally silent during climax while others resemble the Charge of the Light Brigade. It seems a shame to fake orgasm, however, when improved communication with your partner could help you *become* orgasmic. According to experts, foreplay prolonged for a minimum of 20 minutes, plus intercourse sustained for 15 minutes, allows 98% of women to climax eventually. Interestingly, coital orgasm remains elusive for many women until several years after first making love.

SEX

A woman may feel driven to fake an orgasm to 'win' the battle of the sexes, to demonstrate the quality of a relationship by the achievement of 'simultaneous' orgasm – or simply to get things over with.

Eight per cent of women have never achieved orgasm (are 'anorgasmic'), even when masturbating. Psychosexual therapy forms a successful route to becoming orgasmic in many cases. Anorgasmic females are given a series of 'exercises' to perform at home – exploring their own anatomy, learning to communicate needs to partners and learning to accept and give non-penetrative pleasure. Often, intercourse is totally banned. This takes the must-achieve-an-orgasm 'end-point' pressure away and allows relaxation. Referral is via your GP.

3. What should I know about orgasms?

Orgasms rarely last more than 15 seconds. Orgasm itself consists of an intensely pleasurable sensation variously described as emanating from the head, the clitoris, vagina or 'everywhere'. It is accompanied in the female by five to eight major muscle contractions followed by several smaller ones. Nerve impulses spread via the pudendal nerves and cause contraction of the pelvic floor muscles and sometimes thigh muscles as well. *Resolution* follows, where heart rate, blood pressure and genital blood flow return to normal. There is then a short time (usually several minutes) when further orgasm is impossible. This period tends to be shorter than the male equivalent.

Multiple orgasms are possible in the human female. Experiments show that the more orgasms a woman has, the more she is able to have, and the stronger they become. The classic example is nymphomania. Some women can apparently train themselves to reach 100 orgasms in a single night!

During orgasm, a number of brain chemicals are released: prolactin hormone, phenylethylamine (PEA – also found in chocolate) and endorphin. The latter two are addictive, and withdrawal may result in cravings and mild depression!

Orgasms have been classified as clitoral or vaginal depending on which form of stimulation predominates. Vaginal orgasm may feel less 'focussed' and more diffuse because fewer nerve endings, spread further apart, are involved. Most women require some clitoral stimulation and an emotional input to climax.

According to one survey, 50% of males are moderately concerned if the female doesn't orgasm during sex, while 20% are very concerned – which doesn't say a lot for the other 30%!

4. What is a 'normal' sex drive?

According to surveys, 41% of British couples make love more than three times per week, 35% make love once or twice a week and 15% make love two to three times per month. Nine per cent of couples make love less than this or not at all.

The duration of a relationship is significant. Fifty-three per cent of those together for under three years make love more than three times per week. After four years together, only 26% sustain this. Interestingly, it seems the more one earns, the less one is inclined towards sex – presumably stress and exhaustion are to blame! Thirty-five per cent of women feel that men want sex more than they do themselves. This can cause friction in relationships.

The Mangaians of Polynesia make love on average three times per night, every night until the age of 28. After this, their libido falls and they only make love twice per night. Interestingly, this same race believes the female orgasm has to be learned. If a male cannot teach a female to orgasm successfully, her education is entrusted to a friend until she achieves multiple climaxes.

American couples make love one to four times per week, with the universally popular time being 11 pm, especially at weekends. Research, however, shows the best time for sex is when the sun shines. During darkness, the pineal gland in the brain produces melatonin, a chemical which inhibits ovulation, sperm production and hormones responsible for arousal. Pregnancy, contraceptive sales and outbreaks of sexually transmissible disease all peak during the summer and early autumn!

5. *Am I frigid?*

'Frigidity' implies female 'coldness' and can mean anything from failure of orgasm to inability to allow vaginal penetration (vaginissmus). Twenty-nine per cent of women attending genito-urinary clinics and 10% attending family planning clinics admit to sexual dysfunction but tolerate painful intercourse and vaginissmus without seeking help.

Vaginissmus is a distressing condition involving spasm of vaginal, pelvic and even thigh muscles, which prevents penile penetration. There are several recognised causes; some are psychological, some due to anticipation of pain and some due to actual pain:

- lack of lubrication;
- religious or social indoctrination with 'thou shalt nots' and belief that sex is 'dirty';
- previous experience of sexual violence such as assault or rape;
- traumatic childbirth with resulting discomfort;
- post-menopausal discomfort due to atrophy of tissues, especially the protective clitoral hood;
- homosexual orientation.

'Sensate focussing', also known as 'pleasuring', is a popular form of sex therapy for female frigidity. Initially, penetrative sex is banned and a couple take turns to caress and explore each other via foreplay. Genitals and breasts are excluded until both partners are happy to progress to the next stage of 'genital sensate focussing'. Eventually, sometimes after more than 20 sessions lasting an hour each, simple vaginal penetration without subsequent thrusting may be achieved. Later, thrusting is introduced as well. The message to get across is that sexual dysfunctions shouldn't just be tolerated. Pluck up courage and ask your GP for help.

6. *What is the G-spot?*

The G-spot (named after its discoverer, Ernst Grafenberg) hit the headlines a few years ago. It's said to be a button-like area of swollen tissue on the anterior wall of the vagina. When stimulated, it supposedly leads to an urge to urinate followed by rapid orgasm. Occasionally, the female may also

SEX

'ejaculate' some mysterious fluid analogous to semen. Sceptics assumed this fluid was urine. Anatomically and physiologically the G-spot remains both elusive and controversial.

A unique study into human copulation involving ultrasound probes recently showed that sexual penetration from behind or the side achieves the most satisfying orgasms for the female. Thinning of the anterior vaginal wall caused by dragging and stretching of tissues during penile thrusting was found to be remarkable. This may involve stimulation of a G-spot, and also explains why some women leak urine while making love.

7. *Is oral sex safe?*

In surveys, over 90% of women admit to indulging in oral sex. *Cosmopolitan* found that 84% of women adored cunnilingus (male stimulating the female) but only 59% were experiencing it. Seventy-seven per cent of responders were happy to perform fellatio (female stimulating male) but up to 20% didn't actually enjoy it.

Sexually transmissible diseases that can be contracted during oral sex include: herpes, gonorrhoea, candida (thrush), chlamydia (NSU – Non-Specific Urethritis), syphilis and HIV.

The HIV virus has been isolated from saliva, vaginal secretions and semen. During fellatio, those that allow ejaculation of semen into their mouth are at moderate to high risk of HIV transmission. Risk of catching HIV via saliva alone is probably small.

Any bleeding from the gums or vagina (for example sores, menstruation) can potentially pass on infection. Some experts recommend mouth-to-genital contact is avoided unless you definitely know your partner is HIV negative. If you do indulge, the partner performing oral sex should refrain from brushing their teeth beforehand as this can cause gum bleeding. Condoms or dental dams (bubble-gum flavoured latex squares placed over the female genitalia) are essential outside of a long-term relationship – though be careful not to puncture either with your teeth.

8. *Is anal sex normal?*

According to latest research, anal intercourse may be a normal part of heterosexual activity. As many as one in eight teenagers in one survey claim to have experienced it – of whom over 70% of males and 25% of females wished to try it again. The number of adult women regularly participating in anal sex remains constant at approximately 10% – though up to three times as many have tried it and decided it's not for them.

Lubricants are usually used, and sometimes a dilator. Condoms should always be worn.

If you do participate in anal intercourse, be aware of the risks. Firstly, it's illegal – even between man and wife, though the likelihood of being caught and prosecuted seems slim.

Always be hygiene-wise. Bowel bacteria readily cause cystitis and vaginal infections. After anal sex, make sure your partner washes his fingers and penis and changes condoms before any subsequent vaginal contact.

SEX

Rectal sex is a very high risk activity for transmission of HIV – one reason why the gay community has been affected. Rectal intercourse causes abnormal dilatation of anal sphincter muscles. This disrupts lining cells and can result in bleeding. In addition, viral absorption across delicate rectal tissues seems to occur very readily. Because so many bacteria are present in faeces, it's possible that natural defence mechanisms are different in the rectum compared to the vagina. This may in some way allow or even enhance HIV virus transmission.

9. Is masturbation harmful?

Over 90% of healthy adults masturbate, even those who are married and have a happy sex life. Many couples include masturbation (self- as well as mutual stimulation) as a regular part of foreplay. It is not harmful, except psychologically when associated with feelings of guilt and shame. If males masturbate more than three times a day, swelling of the lymph drainage system in the penis may result in a raised, white lump called a 'lymphocoele' (this can also happen if sexual intercourse is frequent). This disappears with a few days' abstinence. Women who overdo DIY stimulation may find vulval tissues become congested enough for orgasmic contractions to be unpleasant and cramping. Again, abstinence relieves the condition.

10. What happens to sperm inside me?

Spermatozoa ascend the female genital tract unless stopped by a barrier method of contraception. Their mission is to search out attractant chemicals secreted by a newly-released oocyte (egg). Millions of sperm are deposited in the vagina, but only 50–100 actually get as far as the egg – usually in the outer half of the fallopian tube; the rest die. Some are absorbed by scavenger cells (macrophages) on the vaginal epithelium and broken down. Others are wafted downwards by a combination of gravity, wave-like motions of cell surfaces (cilia), muscular contractions and eddy currents, to be excreted with vaginal fluids. A few sperm reach the end of the fallopian tubes and enter the abdominal cavity. Here, they will be engulfed by macrophages without causing harm. Sperm can survive alive inside the female tract for up to five days, although fertilising ability is usually lost after 48 hours. This has implications for contraceptive practice.

11. *What are the symptoms and signs of sexually transmitted diseases?*

These vary. Often an infected woman may notice nothing unusual. In general, the following are good indications that you should request a genito-urinary check-up:

- changes in your usual vaginal discharge (increased quantity, unusual smell, unusual colour-staining);
- itch;
- soreness, tenderness, or pain;
- painful intercourse;
- abnormal bleeding;
- lumps;
- ulceration;
- pain on urinating (for example cystitis);
- genital problems in your regular partner;

SEX

- unprotected sex (sex without condoms) with a new partner, especially if abroad.

Symptoms sometimes don't occur until infection is advanced (for example chlamydia). If you suspect you may have a sexually transmitted disease, seek help sooner rather than later.

HIV may show itself as a non-specific glandular-fever-like illness. This is commonly reported in Australia but for some reason is rarely diagnosed in the UK. This acute illness occurs two to six weeks after infection and consists of fever, sore throat, lethargy and joint pains. Glands (lymph nodes) may be enlarged. Sometimes a non-specific 'viral' rash occurs on the trunk and upper limbs. Only a high index of suspicion is likely to lead to an early diagnosis of this condition.

Other presentations of HIV and Aids include: recurrent 'minor' infections (for example oral thrush, skin fungi, persistent herpes); hairy leukoplakia (white, hairy-looking plaques on the tongue or inner cheek); Kaposi's sarcoma – a purplish-red form of cancer involving small blood vessels on the skin or internal organs. Occasionally the first inkling of the disease may be a sudden, serious illness such as pneumonia.

12. How common are HIV and Aids?

Acquired Immune Deficiency Syndrome first appeared in the UK in 1982. Latest figures show that diagnosis of Aids is on the increase, with 380 new cases recognised in the quarter up to the end of December 1992, This brings the cumulative UK

WHAT WORRIES WOMEN MOST

total to 6929. Sadly, of these, over sixty per cent (4291) have already died, of whom 230 were women. On average, another ten victims die each week. All but a few are in groups associated with high risk or high risk behaviour (homosexuals; drug users; haemophiliacs; those transfused with infected blood; those having unprotected sex with high risk partners, especially abroad; babies infected by HIV-positive mothers).

19,065 people are known to be HIV positive in the UK by December 1992, but there may be ten times this number who are undiagnosed and unaware of their status. Seventy-one per cent of Aids cases and sixty-three per cent of HIV cases were reported in the London area.

Worldwide, there are at least 13 million HIV-positive humans and it is estimated that one new case occurs every 15–20 seconds. The World Health Organisation predicts that there will be 40 million affected by the year 2000. Computer models show the number of people infected could double every three years.

In Thailand, 90% of child prostitutes are HIV positive within two years of being forced into the profession. Few use condoms. All street prostitutes in Kenya are HIV positive and many have co-existent ulcerating conditions (syphilis, herpes, and other exotic STDs not usually found in Britain) which increase the risk of HIV transmission.

In the USA, at least a million people are infected with HIV. In New York, Aids is the commonest cause of death in young women and it has been estimated that during 1991, an Aids victim died every 12 minutes; these are sobering figures indeed.

SEX

In December 1992, the US Center for Disease Control changed the definition of Aids to include those who are HIV positive and also have low blood counts of the immune helper cell wiped out by HIV. This will increase diagnosed Aids cases in the US by about 160,000. The current number of reported victims is in the region of 250,000.

Due to improved treatment, the average survival time for patients with full-blown Aids has increased from 10 months to 20 months during the last three years.

13. Can heterosexual sex pass on HIV?

Most people who are HIV positive have indulged in high-risk behaviour (see above) or had unsafe sex with an at-risk partner. However, HIV infection as a result of heterosexual intercourse in the UK has risen by twenty-six per cent during the past year according to the Public Health Laboratory Service. Heterosexual sex now accounts for many new UK cases. *Don't panic* – the majority of new infections involve unsafe sex with obviously risky partners, as the following study shows.

Of 491 Aids cases diagnosed in Britain in the quarter up to March 1992, 55 had slept with bisexuals and drug abusers; 391 had sexual partners who came from countries where Aids is endemic (for example Rwanda, Uganda, Zaire); 63 contracted Aids from unsafe sex abroad; and 5 had strong connections with Africa. Only 47 denied high-risk behaviour, but two were later found to be prostitutes and seven had had contact with prostitutes.

The World Health Organisation has predicted

that by the year 2000, 90% of HIV infections worldwide will be acquired through heterosexual sex – the current estimate is 80%. It is important to remember that the majority of heterosexual spread occurs abroad – Africa, Asia, South America and the Middle East – in people practising unsafe sex (no condoms) and dangerous sex (unprotected anal intercourse), often as part of a thriving sex industry.

Normal heterosexual sex *in the United Kingdom* is relatively low on the risk list so long as partners – and their previous partners ad infinitum – have not participated in high-risk behaviour. Most new cases are imported from abroad but these days, any risk is a risk not worth taking. Safer sex is worth observing. Epidemiologists across Europe have confirmed that male-to-female transmission is twice as likely as the other way round.

14. *What is safer sex?*

The Human Immunodeficiency Virus is transmitted in three main ways:

- sexual contact;
- via blood (transfusion, needles);
- mother to infant before or during birth.

Our main protection against HIV and Aids is through *safer sex*:

- always use strong condoms (certified BS3704) and/or dental dams (see Question 7);
- remember that sex can be pleasurable without penetration. Petting and mutual masturbation are safe providing there is no exchange of body

SEX

fluids (blood, semen). Transmission by saliva is possible but not yet proven;
- never share sex toys (for example vibrators), and always wash them after use;
- avoid enemas or douching, which may scratch or cause inflammation;
- lesbians can catch HIV too. Use dental dams; avoid sex during menstruation; be wary of activities such as fisting, where bleeding can occur; cover cuts on fingers;
- even if both partners are HIV positive, still observe safe sexual practices. Re-infection may further harm your immune system.

Remember that sex, even safer sex, with at-risk partners (for example bisexuals, drug abusers, casual contacts abroad or with those from endemic countries) greatly increases your chances of contracting HIV.

Interestingly, one doctor has suggested that up to 20% of the population are resistant to developing Aids.

15. What are pheromones?

Pheromones are volatile chemicals secreted in very small amounts to affect mood. They are a key to sexual attraction and until recently, had only been isolated in 'lower' animals; for example, the female Chinese silk worm can attract a male up to six miles away.

The first human equivalent has now been isolated – from skin fragments in discarded orthopaedic plaster casts! The discoverer noticed his mood was affected by extracts from this decomposing, sloughed skin. Various liquid concentrates were tested on 40 volunteers, and feelings described as a 'contented high' put pheromone recipients into a friendly, responsive mood. Apparently the pheromone has no detectable smell – despite its smelly origins!

If, as is planned, this pheromone extract is added to perfumes and aftershave, life should shortly prove interesting. Presumably free condoms will be included in every box?

Psychologists suggest nuzzling up to your partner, and sniffing the aroma of fresh, clean skin is one of nature's most powerful tranquillisers. The smell evokes reassuring feelings of love, safety and comfort reminiscent of mothers' arms. Pheromones are probably involved.

16. *Why does sex sometimes hurt?*

Sex can be painful for a woman in several different ways, and this should always be investigated.

Superficial discomfort can result from infection (thrush, bacterial imbalances, chlamydia, trichomonas etc); lack of secretions; rigidity of the hymen; trauma; childbirth (for example episiotomy); other surgery; and psychological problems such as vaginissmus.

Deep pain felt during thrusting actions by the male is commonly due to the penis hitting an ovary. These are just as tender as the male testicles. Experimenting with changes in sexual position may solve the problem. If not, operative tethering of the

SEX

ovary out of the 'line of fire' (using keyhole surgery) may be required.

More serious causes of deep pain during sex include inflammation of the lining of the womb, endometriosis (see Question 62), ectopic pregnancy, fibroids, pelvic inflammatory disease and ovarian masses such as cysts.

CONTRACEPTION AND ABORTION

Contraception has a fascinating history, paying credit to the ingenuity of man (and woman!). From Babylonian crocodile dung to lemon diaphragms, from gold vaginal balls to platinum coils, many modern contraceptives have obvious parallels in ancient times. Even the condom is derived from pouches of sheep intestine and intricately embroidered leather – though its role was more to protect against the ravages of venereal disease than to prevent unwanted pregnancy.

The most fascinating analogue is of the pill: nubile ladies in ancient China swallowed tadpoles in an attempt to prevent unwanted pregnancy. If this failed, they swallowed bees the following year!

The following table gives an idea of the popularity of each method of contraception in Great Britain (1989).

METHOD	% USE
Oral contraceptive pill	25
IUCD (coil)	6
Condom	16
Diaphragm	1
Withdrawal	4
Rhythm method	2
Female sterilisation	11
Male sterilisation	12
No method	28

5% of people hedged their bets and used two methods.

CONTRACEPTION AND ABORTION

Most forms of contraception only fail due to human error. We forget to take a pill, handle a sheath with scissor-like finger nails or remove a diaphragm too early.

The following table shows how effective various methods of contraception are *with careful use:*

METHOD	USER EFFICACY
Coitus Interruptus	83%
Natural Methods	80–98%
Spermicides alone	85%
The Sponge	75%
Male Sheath	85–98%
Female Sheath	85–98%
Diaphragm + spermicide	85–98%
Coil (IUCD)	97–99%
Combined Pill	99%
Mini-Pill	96–99%
Morning-After Pill	96–99%
Morning-After IUCD	99.9%
Depot Progestogen Injection	99%
Sterilisation	99.9%

(1 in 1000 vasectomies fail)
(1–3 female sterilisations fail per 1000)
NB Oil-based products such as petroleum jelly and baby oil can dissolve the rubber of condoms and caps. Tests show condom strength may be reduced by up to 95% within 15 minutes!

17. *How does the combined pill work?*

The combined pill contains two hormones (an oestrogen and a progestogen) which are taken once a day for three weeks. Seven pill-free days follow in

WHAT WORRIES WOMEN MOST

which a light 'withdrawal' bleed, similar to a period, occurs. You are still protected against pregnancy during this pill-free week as long as no pills from the packet on either side are missed.

The combined pill acts by inhibiting ovulation. It mimics the feedback effect on the brain of hormones secreted during pregnancy. This switches off brain secretion of other hormones (FSH – follicle stimulating hormone and LH – luteinising hormone) necessary for the growth and maturation of eggs.

Progestogens provide extra contraceptive protection by several secondary actions: they thicken cervical mucus so that sperm cannot penetrate; the lining of the womb becomes thin and less receptive to implantation of a fertilised egg; the transport of eggs and sperm in the fallopian tube is impaired so that eggs and sperm migrate less easily.

Women over 35 who smoke should use an alternative method of contraception. Smoking and the pill jointly increase the stickiness of blood, and the risk of serious side-effects in smokers increases with age. Non-smokers can be reassured that modern low-dose pills may be taken safely right up until the menopause. Most doctors now feel the low dosage pills are perfectly safe for women over 35.

Possible unwanted side-effects of the combined pill include nausea, headache, mood changes, breast tenderness, weight gain, breakthrough bleeding, jaundice, thrombosis, raised blood pressure and stroke.

CONTRACEPTION AND ABORTION

18. How does the mini-pill work?

The mini-pill contains only one type of hormone (a progestogen) and is taken consecutively every day without a tablet-free break. Periods come when they want to – and in some women disappear altogether (see below). Most bleeds occurring while taking the mini-pill are light and regular.

The mini-pill doesn't necessarily inhibit ovulation. Eggs may be released in the middle of a cycle but fertilisation doesn't occur, as the mini-pill exerts the same progestogen effects as the combined pill: thickened cervical mucus, thinned womb lining and decreased tubal motility. Together, these form the basis for contraceptive protection.

The mini-pill is less reliable than the combined pill and should be taken within three hours of the correct time every day. If delayed, cervical mucus starts to liquefy and contraceptive protection may be lost. Some users find a programmable alarm watch useful to remind them when their mini-pill is due.

Possible unwanted side-effects of the mini-pill include menstrual irregularity, spotting and absence of periods (amenorrhoea). Lack of periods is not harmful so long as pregnancy can be excluded: it implies that ovulation has been inhibited. Some women are uneasy with absent periods, and prefer to change to a different type of progestogen so that menstruation returns.

WHAT WORRIES WOMEN MOST

19. *What should I do if I forget to take a combined pill?*

It's important to avoid lengthening the 7-day pill-free interval. Contrary to popular belief, ovulation is more likely to occur if the first or last pills in a pack are forgotten rather than the pills in the middle. During the pill-free week, egg follicles often start developing but are damped down when pill-taking restarts. Any pills missed on either side of the pill-free break allow follicle development to progress, and increase the risk that an egg will ripen and be released.

If your combined pill is less than 12 hours overdue, don't panic. Just take the delayed pill NOW and resume normal pill-taking when the next dose is due.

If your pill is more than 12 hours delayed:

(i) take the delayed pill *now* and resume normal pill-taking when the next one is due;
(ii) use extra precautions (for example condoms) for the next seven days;
(iii) count how many pills are left in your pack after the delayed pill. If *seven or more* pills remain, leave the usual break after this pack before starting your next pack. If *fewer than seven* pills remain, start a new pack the day *after* finishing this one – that is, don't have your usual seven-day break or period.

If two or more pills have been missed, especially from the first five at the start of the packet, it's worth considering the 'morning-after pill'. Seek the advice

CONTRACEPTION AND ABORTION

of your doctor on whether you are at risk of pregnancy. You may be advised not to take any more pills until pregnancy has been ruled out.

20. What should I do if I forget to take a mini-pill?

There's very little room for manoeuvre here. The mini-pill's effect on penetrability of cervical mucus to sperm is greatest four hours after ingestion and wears off during the next 24 hours. Therefore, if a mini-pill is only three hours late (that is, 27 hours after the last tablet), extra precautions should be started *immediately* and used for the next *seven* days. Until recently, guidelines only recommended 48 hours' worth of additional protection, but this is now thought not to be long enough.

If two or more pills have been missed, the morning-after pill should be considered.

21. How long after unprotected sex does the morning-after pill work?

The morning-after pill is more flexible than it sounds and can be started within 72 hours of unprotected sex. The most popular method, the Yuzpe method, involves taking two tablets as soon as possible (within the 72 hour limit), then taking two more 12 hours later – even if this means setting the alarm and waking in the middle of the night. This regime can make you very sick and is not guaranteed to work (up to a 4% failure rate). One advantage is that women usually bleed within three

WHAT WORRIES WOMEN MOST

weeks of taking the morning-after pill and therefore have 'proof' that it has worked. They can then resume their normal method of contraception. Women who don't bleed should have a pregnancy test.

Hormonal methods of emergency contraception work by:

- rendering the womb lining unfavourable for implantation;
- upsetting the transportation of the ovum down the fallopian tubes.
- preventing or delaying ovulation if given early enough;
- altering the hormone secreting function of the corpus luteum – the name given to the ovarian follicle which creates the hormones necessary to continue a pregnancy.

22. What other methods of emergency contraception are available?

The coil can be inserted *in good faith* as an emergency form of contraception up to five days after the earliest possible calculation of ovulation (using a woman's menstrual dates) following unprotected sex. In practice, this is usually interpreted as up to five days from the sexual act itself.

Other hormones are being researched as post-coital contraceptives, including progestogens and the newly available anti-progesterone mifepristone (RU486) – coined the 'abortion drug'. World Health Organisation data suggests mifepristone is very effective in that no one who took it during trials got

CONTRACEPTION AND ABORTION

pregnant and it caused little nausea and vomiting. A disadvantage is that it sometimes delays the next period so a woman will worry that she has conceived after all.

Strictly speaking, purists would regard methods of emergency contraception as abortion-inducing agents. The modern view, upheld in court, is that fertilisation is a process starting with the fertilisation of an egg but not completed until implantation has occurred. The term 'emergency contraception' is therefore justifiable. This is an intensely personal moral and ethical area. It is essential that full information and counselling takes place before emergency contraception is used. Any woman with doubts about the acceptability of her chosen form of contraception should express these to her family planning specialist.

If emergency contraception fails, exposure to hormones is unlikely to cause abnormality of the foetus; induced abortion is therefore not considered necessary for medical reasons.

Needless to say, no woman should ever rely on emergency forms of contraception as their sole method.

23. *Is inserting a diaphragm easy?*

Like everything else, practice makes perfect. Many women introduced to the diaphragm for the first time when aged 35–40 years (for example after stopping the pill) are surprised at how easy it is to use. The diaphragm (or cap) is a thin, latex dome with a flexible, spring-loaded rim. It is designed to cover the cervix and stays in place by a combination

WHAT WORRIES WOMEN MOST

of the vaginal muscles, the spring-loaded tension of the ring and the pubic bone. Your correct size (between 50 and 100 mm in diameter) must first be determined by a trained practitioner. If your weight changes by more than half a stone (3 kg) the fitting of your cap should be re-checked.

Diaphragms should always be used with a recommended spermicide or they lose maximum contraceptive potential. They can be inserted either way up, but maintain the correct position more readily if inserted dome upwards.

Squirt spermicide around the rim on the upper surface of the dome and in two parallel lines over the top of the dome. Some women find foam preparations easier to use and direct.

Insert the diaphragm before making love and leave in place for six hours after the last intercourse – otherwise sperm might still ascend the cervical canal. Use extra spermicide for each act of intercourse *and* if you make love for the first time more than three hours after insertion.

When inserting the diaphragm, make sure your bladder is empty and adopt the position you find most comfortable for inserting a tampon.

With an index finger inside the rim of the cap, gently compress the rim between your thumb and remaining fingers, with the spermicide-coated dome pointing upwards. With the other hand, gently separate the labia and insert the diaphragm inwards and backwards. Tuck the front rim of the cap up behind your pubic bone, where it should fit snugly and comfortably. Insert your index finger and check that your cervix (which feels like a rubber cone) is fully covered.

CONTRACEPTION AND ABORTION

The diaphragm pulls out by hooking your index finger (plus middle finger if preferred) behind the front rim and pulling downwards and outwards. Don't leave a diaphragm in place for longer than 24 hours, as this both encourages infection and gives a theoretical risk of pressure damage to vaginal walls.

24. How does the contraceptive injection work?

Contraceptive injections contain micro-crystalline suspensions of progestogen. They are given once every 12 weeks into the buttock and the hormone is slowly and continuously released. The injection works in a similar way to the mini-pill, but also inhibits ovulation.

The injection is currently licensed for use in women for whom other contraceptives are considered inadvisable for medical reasons, for example because they have caused unacceptable side-effects. This would include, for example, those who cannot remember to take their pill or those requiring foolproof contraception while their partner undergoes a vasectomy. The main reported side-effects are menstrual disturbances such as irregular periods, spotting between periods or complete absence of periods. Some users experience weight gain, headaches, fluid retention or mood changes.

Progestogen preparations are proving increasingly acceptable – hence the development of several new forms (see Question 27).

WHAT WORRIES WOMEN MOST

25. *Is sterilisation really irreversible?*

Any couple considering sterilisation should assume this method is irreversible. In practice, advances in surgical techniques mean reversal of vasectomy achieves pregnancy in 40% of cases following microsurgery and 30% of cases where traditional surgery is used.

Reversal of female sterilisation entails major abdominal surgery and a resultant scar. It has a 50% success rate but the risks, including pelvic infection or fertilisation taking place outside the womb (ectopic pregnancy), are great.

26. *Can you get pregnant during a period?*

Yes, if adequate contraception is not being used. There are recorded cases of conception on every day of the menstrual cycle – including the actual period – resulting from isolated acts of intercourse. Sometimes an egg is released at an unpredictable and unusual time in the cycle. Sperm remain viable in the female tract for up to five days and are capable of fertilising an egg for at least two days, probably longer.

27. *What new forms of contraception are being developed?*

Due to the side-effects associated with oestrogen, some experts feel progesterone-only methods of contraception are the way forward. Progestogen capsules surgically implanted under the skin,

CONTRACEPTION AND ABORTION

progestogen-impregnated vaginal rings and a progestogen-enhanced coil are likely to become available in the UK during 1993–94.

Future methods of contraception are likely to involve nasal sprays which will switch fertility 'on' or 'off' at will. A male contraceptive pill with acceptable side-effects is still being sought – as is a vas deferens 'tap' in the tube cut during a vasectomy, to control the release of sperm into seminal fluid.

28. *What are the legal requirements for termination of pregnancy?*

To conform with the Human Fertilisation and Embryology Act 1990 and the Abortion Act 1967, two doctors must agree that one of the following grounds for termination are present:

A. the continuance of the pregnancy would involve risk to the life of the pregnant woman greater than if the pregnancy were terminated;
B. the termination is necessary to prevent grave permanent injury to the physical or mental health of the pregnant woman;
C. the pregnancy has NOT exceeded its 24th week, and the continuance of the pregnancy would involve risk, greater than if the pregnancy were terminated, of injury to the physical or mental health of the pregnant woman;
D. the pregnancy has NOT exceeded its 24th week and the continuance of the pregnancy would involve risk, greater than if the pregnancy were terminated, of injury to the physical and mental

WHAT WORRIES WOMEN MOST

health of any existing child(ren) of the family of the pregnant woman;
E. there is a substantial risk that if the child were born it would suffer from such physical or mental abnormalities as to be seriously handicapped.

Grounds A, B and E in effect have no time limit. Note that babies born from 24 weeks onwards have survived.

29. What happens during termination of pregnancy?

Initially you will receive counselling to ensure termination is the right decision for you. The procedure used during termination depends on the length of time since conception. The earlier a termination can be carried out, the safer it is – and the less distressing for all those involved.

Suction termination of pregnancy (STOP) can be performed up to 12 weeks as an out-patient under local or general anaesthetic.

After 12 weeks the products of conception are larger and the walls of the womb softer – so perforation can easily complicate the procedure. A mini-labour is therefore usually induced first with vaginal pessaries inserted into the vagina. Medical abortion is rarely complete and a surgical scrape (D & C – dilation and curettage) of retained products routinely follows.

If pregnancy is particularly advanced (for example in the case of foetal abnormality), prostaglandins (hormones) are injected into the amniotic fluid

CONTRACEPTION AND ABORTION

which surrounds the baby along with other chemicals to ensure the foetus is no longer alive on delivery. You will need to be awake during this procedure, which results in greater emotional trauma than earlier methods.

In June 1991, the anti-progesterone abortion pill mifepristone (RU486) was licensed for use with women whose dates are certain or have been confirmed by ultrasound. Mifepristone can only be used during the first nine weeks of pregnancy and is highly effective.

A mifepristone tablet is administered orally in hospital and the woman observed for two hours before going home. She is re-admitted 36–48 hours later, when a prostaglandin pessary is inserted. Abortion usually occurs four to eight hours later.

The two main side-effects of this treatment are bleeding and pain – the bleeding persists for 12 days on average.

A decision to go ahead with termination is rarely easy and should only proceed after full counselling. Medical personnel will treat you sympathetically at every step of the way. However, there are significant risks of infection, infertility, and long-lasting emotional trauma as a result of an abortion. The earlier a decision to terminate is made, the safer and less unpleasant the physical and emotional effects will be.

PERIODS

Many myths surround the process of menstruation. In some cultures, periods are even considered taboo. Balinese women are barred from entering temples whilst bleeding and 'sniffer' dogs are trained to 'flush' them out! So ingrained is the idea that menstruating women are possessed by devils that the Polynesian word for periods is *tabu*, which also means 'sacred' and 'unclean'!

In a recent national opinion poll, it was found that most UK women are reluctant to consult their GP for period problems. Ninety per cent of women questioned admitted to suffering dreadfully with their periods, but four out of five resorted to pain-killers, self-help remedies, or suffered in silence until symptoms subsided. Only 18% had sought help from their GP.

There are many causes of painful, heavy periods. If you're having trouble with yours, don't be afraid to seek help. Many modern treatments are available – from both complementary and traditional medicine.

30. *What is a normal menstrual cycle?*

Few women are blessed with a 'normal' menstrual cycle. Textbooks suggest periods occur every 28 days, last five days and result in a blood loss of around 30 ml (two tablespoonsful). Scientific evidence however, suggests a much larger degree of variability within a 'normal' cycle.

Studies have shown periods lasting from two to 18

PERIODS

days, with the commonest length being five to six days. A 'heavy' period lasting over ten days may require treatment.

The famous 28-day lunar cycle of menstruation occurs in only 12% of women. The normal range seems to vary from 15 to over 50 days. Cycle length also varies in the same woman according to her age. On average, the menstrual cycle is longest at puberty and again later as the menopause approaches. It is shortest around the age of 43 years.

The prehistoric cave-woman probably experienced no more than 50 menstrual bleeds during her relatively short life. Mostly she was pregnant or actively breast-feeding. In evolutionary terms, it is possibly normal for us to now experience 400–500 periods during our fertile span. We can blame this on effective contraception!

Periods cause many women to experience pain, inconvenience, distress, anxiety and days off work. If your periods are problematic, help your doctor by keeping a chart like the one below. If you experience post-menopausal bleeding, bleeding after sex or between periods, seek medical assessment immediately.

MENSTRUAL ANALYSIS CHART

Mark the chart on days when symptoms trouble you. Use the symbols below. Start the first month on the first day of your period (day 1) and start a new line for each period.

WHAT WORRIES WOMEN MOST

DAYS OF CYCLE

Month   1 2 3 4 5 6 7 8 9 10 11 12 13 14 15 16 17 18 19 20 21 22 23 24 25 26 27 28 29 . . . (number to the end of your cycle)

I

II

III

X = Period   S = Spotting   P = Pain   D = Depression   I = Irritability   T = Tiredness
B = Bloating   W = Weight gain   O = Breast pain   ! = Intercourse

PERIODS

31. Why are my periods heavy?

Five to ten per cent of women will have heavy vaginal bleeding at some time during their lives. A heavy period (menorrhagia) lasts ten days or longer, with flooding and possibly clots. Anaemia may result.

Tests where tampons and sanitary pads have been weighed show that the number of 'mopper-uppers' used bears little relation to the total quantity of blood lost. Menorrhagia officially occurs when blood loss is greater than 80 ml. Sixty per cent of women complaining of excessive bleeding actually have a blood loss within normal limits. However, it does help your doctor to know how many boxes of pads and tampons you are getting through.

Eighty per cent of heavy bleeds occur when an egg fails to develop during the menstrual cycle. This is common early in life, when periods have just started, and again later, as the menopause approaches. Without ovulation, the second half of the cycle (progesterone secretion) fails to occur. Overstimulation with oestrogen results and the lining of the womb increases and thickens so there is more to shed than normal.

In teenagers, heavy bleeding eventually sorts itself out. If interfering with lifestyle, it can be helped by hormone treatments such as a progestogen or the pill.

In menopausal women, hormone treatment does not always work and it is usually advisable to have a D & C (dilation and curettage or 'scrape') so that trimmings from the womb lining can be examined

WHAT WORRIES WOMEN MOST

microscopically. More serious conditions need to be discounted before treatment is recommended.

Causes of menorrhagia include:

- fibroids – blood loss is often heavy but regular;
- the contraceptive coil (IUCD) – causes heavy, cramping periods;
- polyps – fleshy, benign growths of the womb lining or cervix which can cause 'spotting' between periods or just before a period;
- pelvic inflammatory disease – often causes pain during intercourse as well;
- endometriosis.

Causes of heavy bleeding which need to be discounted are:

- cancers of the cervix, endometrium and ovary;
- pregnancy and miscarriage;
- thyroid and pituitary gland problems;
- blood-clotting disorders.

Women under the age of 35 who experience menorrhagia are unlikely to have a serious disease – but should still consult their doctor. The chance of endometrial cancer in this age group is only one in 100,000.

32. *Why are my periods painful?*

Pain during menstruation (dysmenorrhoea) usually starts with the onset of bleeding and lasts for between several hours and several days. It is spasmodic in nature and may be accompanied by diarrhoea, nausea and even vomiting.

The lining of the womb secretes hormones called

PERIODS

prostaglandins – so named because they were first discovered in the prostate gland. They cause uterine muscles to contract and result in cramping pains. They may also stimulate the gut to produce diarrhoea. Non-steroidal anti-inflammatory drugs such as paracetamol, ibuprofen or mefenamic acid help to stop the cramping pains. Hormone therapy (for example the pill) also helps by preventing congestion of the endometrium.

Self-help regimes that have transformed suffering in many women include aromatherapy, relaxation techniques, hypnosis, acupuncture, and a wholefood, low-salt diet.

Other types or causes of dysmenorrhoea include:

- 'functional' – where no physical cause is found and anti-prostaglandin medication doesn't help. (Some doctors believe this is due to psychosomatic or psychosexual causes – though with sex education this is becoming less common);
- endometriosis;
- fibroids;
- pelvic inflammatory disease;
- contraceptive coils – which can provoke both menorrhagia and dysmenorrhoea.

33. Why are my periods irregular?

Irregular periods may have frequent cycles of 14 days or come infrequently every two to three months. Sometimes they stop altogether.

The commonest causes of infrequent periods are pregnancy, being overweight or significantly underweight, thyroid disease, stress, polycystic ovaries, hormonal contraception, stopping the pill, general illness, and various hormone imbalances. Frequent periods tend to have the same origins as menorrhagia (heavy periods).

Even if your periods aren't heavy or painful, irregularity may indicate an underlying condition needing investigation, for example an under-active or over-active thyroid or a problem with hormone secretion. All cases are therefore worth bringing to your doctor's attention.

34. What will my doctor do if I consult her/him about my periods?

Your doctor will first ask a series of questions to ascertain exactly what's wrong. It will help if you keep a menstrual chart such as suggested in Question 30. Your doctor will then decide whether to perform an internal examination or not. If you are bleeding heavily and prefer to postpone this, don't worry. The 'internal' and a cervical smear, if needed, can be done at a later date. In the meantime, a general examination – including gently feeling your abdomen – will suffice. Your doctor will be checking for anaemia, signs of ill-health (sallowness, weight loss, fingernail changes), distribution and amount of body hair, and appearance of secondary sexual characteristics which develop at puberty. Examining the abdomen will reveal any obvious masses (ovarian cysts, uterine fibroids) and areas of marked tenderness.

Blood tests may be taken to exclude anaemia and check various hormone levels. You may also be asked to take a pregnancy test (see Question 43).

PERIODS

Ideally, an internal examination is required before reaching a diagnosis, prescribing a treatment or referring you to a gynaecologist. In rare cases where a woman is unable to submit to an internal examination, it may prove appropriate to do this under a short-duration general anaesthetic or to perform an ultrasound test of the pelvis instead.

35. What is Toxic Shock Syndrome?

Toxic Shock Syndrome (TSS) is a rare but serious condition often resulting in death. It is associated with two virulent bacteria – which infect the vagina and produce poisons that enter the bloodstream.

Infection is encouraged by drying out and cracking of the vaginal walls, caused by leaving super-absorbent tampons in place too long. The warm, blood-soaked tampon also acts as a fertile breeding ground for bugs.

If virulent bacteria are present, they rapidly enter the bloodstream and produce toxins in a process known as septicaemia (blood poisoning). This rapidly leads to circulatory collapse (shock) and death if not vigorously treated. Occasionally, only mild illness develops, characterised by fever and a rash.

From the beginning of 1993, strong warnings about TSS will appear on packets of tampons, together with inserts describing the condition. In order to prevent toxic shock syndrome, use the tampon with the lowest absorbency possible and change tampons frequently.

Best advice is not to use tampons overnight – this keeps them in place for an unacceptably long time.

What Worries Women Most

If necessary, resort to wearing maternity pads instead.

Always consult your doctor if menstrual blood loss seems excessive.

PRE-MENSTRUAL SYNDROME

Pre-menstrual syndrome is a common and distressing problem affecting over 50% of menstruating women. Twenty to forty per cent of women suffer symptoms severe enough to seek help from their doctor, and 6% are totally incapacitated.

For diagnosis, there must be a clear-cut relationship between symptoms and the menstrual cycle. Problems start in the 14 days before a period and cease promptly when bleeding occurs. A symptom-free phase lasting at least seven consecutive days after menstruation helps distinguish PMS from 'menstrual magnification' – that is, worsening of pre-existing emotional or physical problems before a period. A symptom diary kept for at least two menstrual cycles will therefore assist in making a diagnosis.

Trials of PMS treatments invariably show a strong initial placebo effect (subjective improvement with no active ingredient, from the Latin *placebo* – I please). One study involving surgically implanted hormones showed an amazing 94% of women improved on placebo alone. Unfortunately, this led some researchers to suppose PMS is totally psychosomatic.

36. What are the symptoms of PMS and what causes them?

Symptoms vary in severity from cycle to cycle. More than 150 have been described, including depression, mood swings, anxiety, aggression, irritability, restlessness, tiredness, bingeing, bloating, breast tenderness, poor concentration, loss of self-control, headache and backache. Sex drive (libido) is usually reduced.

In some cases, PMS is so severe the personality of the sufferer changes. Suicide attempts are more frequent in the fortnight before a period, and the incidence of accidents in the home and on the road increases. Crimes such as shoplifting and even murder may occur, but courts have allowed a plea of diminished responsibility if PMS is excessive. Interestingly, men are late for work more often when their partner is pre-menstrual!

The cause of pre-menstrual syndrome remains unclear. Many theories, including dietary, environmental, social, psychological, hormonal and genetic, have been suggested. PMS stops during pregnancy and at the menopause. Many women have benefited from the pill, but it is not always successful.

Hormonal events in the second half of the menstrual cycle probably play a role in PMS, as symptoms do not occur in the absence of ovulation. However, the issue was recently confused by a study in which the luteal phase of hormone events (occurring in the two weeks prior to menstruation) was shortened. The anti-progesterone, mifepristone (the

PRE-MENSTRUAL SYNDROME

abortion pill RU486) and HCG were used to induce early menstruation. Surprisingly, symptoms of PMS showed the same time course and severity, regardless of whether the balance between progesterone and oestrogen was usual for the second half of a normal menstrual cycle or not.

Some doctors believe a relative deficiency of natural progesterone is to blame; others claim there is insufficient evidence to back this theory up. Latest research shows that PMS may be due to an inability of progesterone receptors to bind progesterone hormone (see next question).

37. *What treatments are available for PMS?*

The most effective treatments seem to be those which totally suppress ovulation, such as the pill.

Oil of evening primrose, regular exercise, and reducing dietary caffeine, alcohol, sugar, additives and salt, are all said to help. Vitamin B6 is popular but is dangerous if an overdose is taken, and can cause abnormality in the foetus; long-term treatment, especially with doses exceeding 200 mg per day, is not recommended.

Many PMS sufferers have found relief from relaxation training, aromatherapy, homeopathy and acupuncture. Hormone treatment (for example skin patches, hormone implants, the anti-oestrogen bromocriptine) to suppress ovulation is recommended if simpler treatments fail.

Some doctors recommend treatment with progesterone pessaries to correct a theoretical imbalance.

WHAT WORRIES WOMEN MOST

This works in prophylaxis, but not once symptoms have started. Latest research shows that progesterone-binding receptors may be at fault – they don't bind progesterone efficiently when adrenaline hormone is present. Adrenaline is released when blood glucose levels reach a critically low level. Nibbling regular carbohydrate snacks (such as digestive biscuits) raises blood sugar and enhances progesterone-receptor binding, which may explain the cravings and bingeing which often occur during PMS.

Adopting a three-hourly starch diet (flour, potatoes, oats, rice or rye) may relieve or even cure symptoms by keeping blood sugar levels raised. In one famous trial, relief from symptoms was obtained on this regime in 89% of women suffering true PMS. Of those with menstrual magnification (non-PMS worsening of another condition), 55% gained some benefit. Dietary manipulation alone, with no additional medication, provided full relief of severe PMS in 19% of sufferers.

If all else fails, research from New Zealand suggests the newer types of antidepressants (which raise levels of a brain chemical, serotonin) reduced PMS in 15 out of 16 women. This data must be viewed with interest until more information becomes available.

INFERTILITY

It is estimated that in any one year, a million British couples are actively trying for pregnancy. The average chance of conceiving is 20% per month, and most couples will have achieved their objective within one year.

Infertility is the commonest reason for referral to hospital in people under the age of 40. One in 20 males are subfertile or infertile at any one time and 25% of women will experience some form of reduced fertility – one in eight while trying for a first baby. Three per cent of women are involuntarily childless and 6% are unable to have as many children as they would wish.

Modern women often delay motherhood into their 30s and significant numbers have problems conceiving as a result. Fertility declines with age, as can be seen from the following table:

Age of woman	Average time to pregnancy	Monthly chance of pregnancy with artificial insemination
25 years	2–3 months	11%
35 years	6 months or longer	6.5%

There is still a surprising amount of misunderstanding about fertility. A survey sponsored by Carter Wallace in 1991 found that:

- almost half of British men and 39% of women believe the female needs an orgasm to achieve pregnancy;
- 57% of women and 76% of men don't know

WHAT WORRIES WOMEN MOST

that women are most fertile in the middle of the menstrual cycle;
- 17% of women under 24 years old don't know how to confirm they're pregnant;
- 8% of women and 11% of men believe pregnancy should occur within the first month of trying.

38. Why can't I get pregnant?

Subfertility is defined as 'failure to conceive after twelve months of regular intercourse'. Causes of subfertility remain unexplained in 30% of cases despite extensive investigation – but stress plays a significant part. New research indicates that antibodies against sperm, or the absence of enzymes needed by sperm for successful penetration of an ovum, may be at fault.

Male factors are significant in around 19% of cases of subfertility. Female ovulatory failure accounts for 27% of cases, tubal damage for 14% and endometriosis for 5%.

Many couples are often dismissively told to 'try harder'; information about a woman's fertile peak would be more useful. The window of fertility is only 24–36 hours long and usually occurs in the middle of the menstrual cycle. In a regular 28 day cycle, this will centre around day 14, where day 1 is counted as the first day of menstrual bleeding. Using an ovulation prediction kit will maximise chances of pregnancy.

It is important not to make conception the linchpin of your life. A 'laid back' approach is more likely to succeed than a frantic rummage under the sheets

INFERTILITY

to appease the menstrual clock. The following simple tips will assist fertility:

- the scrotum needs to be 4°C cooler than body temperature. Males should wear cotton boxer shorts and loose-fitting trousers. Daily cold water douching of the testicles is recommended by some experts;
- both partners should stop smoking. Smokers are only half as fertile as non-smokers;
- cut out alcohol. Forty per cent of male infertility is linked to moderate alcohol intake. Evidence points to a similar alcohol association in women – it hastens degeneration of eggs in the ovary;
- decrease your consumption of caffeine – a study has shown an impressive link between subfertility and drinking over eight cups of coffee per day;
- supplement your diet with zinc and vitamins E, C and B12;
- improve your general fitness and in particular ensure your weight is in the normal range;
- learn to beat stress with relaxation techniques and try, for example, aromotherapy, homeopathy or acupuncture;
- previously, men were advised to abstain from sex for three days prior to their partner's predicted date of ovulation to maximise chances of pregnancy. If there is difficulty in conceiving, latest research suggests abstinence for seven to ten days may be beneficial.

WHAT WORRIES WOMEN MOST

39. *How are grandmothers able to conceive?*

Pregnancy may occur naturally, though rarely, up to 55 years of age. Recently, women have been helped to give birth over this age. In South Africa, a grandmother acted as surrogate mother for her own daughter and gave birth to triplets – her genetic grandchildren; another woman has delivered twins using eggs donated by her best friend. In yet another case to hit the headlines, a 42-year-old American woman bore twins – her own grandchildren – for a daughter who was born without a uterus.

The oldest woman to give birth via assisted conception techniques was 62. In all these cases, eggs were harvested from donors and fertilised *in vitro* (test-tube babies).

The post-menopausal recipient is primed with oestrogen and progestogen hormones on the day before donor eggs are harvested, to make her endometrium receptive to implantation. Further hormones are administered for the first 15 weeks gestation (tablets or injections) after which the placenta is mature enough to maintain the pregnancy itself.

Technically, this process is easier than implanting fertilised eggs into pre-menopausal women who are still menstruating. Synchronisation of hormone cycles is then required between donor and recipient.

In one controversial twist which has upset both clergy and lawyers alike, a 19-year-old Italian girl has acted as a surrogate for her own mother – and given birth to her genetic brother!

INFERTILITY

40. What tests are done for infertility?

Examination of the infertile couple may reveal anatomical abnormalities such as malformed pelvic organs or varicose veins (varicocoeles) of the scrotum. These varicose veins overheat the testes by 2°C and inactivate sperm. The condition can be corrected surgically or the veins sealed with special injections.

The simplest fertility test is for a woman to take her temperature every morning before getting out of bed. This will go up a fraction of a degree when ovulation occurs. Recently, however, the value of temperature charts has been called into question.

Guidelines recommend initially assessing a woman's blood progesterone levels (other hormone assays are taken as well) on day 21 of the cycle to assess whether ovulation has occurred. If it has, progesterone levels will be high. Simultaneously, semen from her partner can be sent for analysis to save time.

A post-coital test involves sampling cervical mucus the morning after an 'active' night before. This has occasionally brought to light a total misunderstanding of the process of copulation in apparently infertile couples: absence of sperm indicates that the male is infertile – or lack of knowledge of what 'proper' sexual intercourse is about! Present but inactivated sperm may indicate an incompatibility problem such as anti-sperm antibodies.

Ultrasound scanning of the ovaries, dye tests to flush the fallopian tubes and establish patency, laparoscopy (keyhole surgery to visually examine the female reproductive organs via a scope) and occasionally, an examination of womb tissue (endometrial biopsy) may be recommended. A new technique, 'falloposcopy', allows a flexible telescope to be inserted into the fallopian tubes via the uterus. Doctors can then assess the extent of internal scarring (from, for example, previous pelvic inflammatory disease) and determine whether tubal surgery would help. Falloposcopy can also clear the uterine end of the tubes of up to 40% obstruction due to debris.

Luteinising Hormone Releasing Hormone (LHRH) is secreted in pulses every one to four hours by one part of the brain (hypothalamus) to stimulate another (the pituitary gland). The pituitary responds by releasing pulses of Follicle Stimulating Hormone (FSH) and Luteinising Hormone (LH) – collectively known as gonadotrophins. FSH usually stimulates the ovary to initiate development of egg follicles. This system can be assessed for responsiveness by injecting LHRH and measuring blood hormone levels over the following hour.

Special testing is required to analyse sperm for the enzyme necessary to penetrate an egg. This technique is only available in a few centres.

41. *What methods are available to help me achieve pregnancy?*

Obviously this depends on the cause of infertility. *In-vitro* (test-tube) fertilisation, with implantation of the resultant fertilised egg into the uterus, has a success rate which varies with maternal age. At 28

INFERTILITY

years, the pregnancy rate per treatment cycle is 22%. At 32 years, it is 15%, and it falls to 9.5% at a maternal age of 40. Miscarriage rates increase with age, so the 'take-home-baby' rate is less.

Fertility drugs stimulate natural hormone production to trigger ovulation, but 'super-ovulation' (producing lots of eggs) and multiple pregnancy are a risk. The drug clomiphene causes ovulation in 75% of eligible women and 35% of these will become pregnant. The risk of twins, however, is 5% (normal incidence is 1¼ per cent).

Human Menopausal Gonadotrophin (HMG; extracted from the urine of post-menopausal women) contains follicle stimulating hormone (FSH) that triggers development of ovarian follicles, and leutinising hormone (LH) which ripens and releases an egg. In women eligible for this treatment, 75–90% will ovulate and 35% will achieve pregnancy. However, the risk of multiple pregnancy (often with six or seven embryos) is 35%. If the majority survive, difficulties can arise on delivery (prematurity, respiratory distress syndrome, cerebral palsy, failure to thrive, etc).

A hormone releasing hormone (LHRH) can be injected into the subcutaneous fat in 'pulses' via a pump to simulate normal release from the brain. This results in 90% of cycles becoming ovulatory and after six months, 90% of patients are pregnant.

Many other treatment advances have been made. GIFT (Gamete Intra-Fallopian Transfer – where test-tube fertilised eggs are flushed into the fallopian tubes) has a success rate of 21% per treatment cycle (multiple pregnancy rate 21%). DIPI (Direct Intra-Peritoneal Insemination) has a success rate of 10%

What Worries Women Most

per treatment cycle; and POST (Peritoneal Oocyte and Sperm Transfer) is successful in 25% of treatment cycles. State-of-the-art techniques have success rates varying from 17 to 37%. These include:

- SUZI – SubZonal Insemination (injection of a single sperm into an egg);
- TUFT – Trans-Uterine Fallopian Transfer;
- TET – Tubal Embryo Transfer;
- PROST – ProNuclear Stage Tubal Transfer;
- ZIFT – Zygote Intra-Fallopian Tube Transfer;

and many more. The message is very much one of hope for couples experiencing infertility.

PREGNANCY

A five-month-old female foetus contains about seven million eggs. By the time of birth, this number falls to two million and by the time of puberty, less than half a million remain. The rest have slowly degenerated and resorbed. No new eggs are ever formed after birth – when we talk about 'making' eggs, we mean maturation of egg cells (ova) already present in the ovary.

Usually, only one egg (ovum) matures fully during each menstrual cycle. Several other follicles will start to grow but only the fastest, 'dominant' ovum is released. The rest fail Darwin's 'survival of the fittest' test and die. Once ovulation occurs, the empty follicle collapses and forms a yellow cyst known as the corpus luteum. This secretes oestrogen and progesterone to switch off further production of FSH and LH in the hypothalamus. If pregnancy occurs, the corpus luteum continues to secrete hormones and maintains early pregnancy by preventing menstruation. After the third month of pregnancy, the placenta takes over and the corpus luteum wanes. If pregnancy doesn't occur, the corpus luteum degenerates after about ten days. This triggers menstruation and the start of a new cycle.

In theory, only one sperm is needed to achieve fertilisation of the ovum. On average, the male deposits 200–300 million sperm into the female tract per ejaculation but only 50–150 eventually reach the egg – usually in the upper half of the fallopian tube. If the concentration of male sperm is consistently

WHAT WORRIES WOMEN MOST

below 20 million per millilitre, the chance of infertility is surprisingly great.

Semen is initially thick and sticky. Within 20–30 minutes it is broken down by enzymes and becomes liquid, and the great sperm race begins. During artificial insemination, it was noted that some very active sperm reach the fallopian tubes within five minutes of being deposited! Some sperm, however, remain in the cervical mucus 'plug' for several days, with a constant stream swimming up into the uterus and tubes.

Once a sperm penetrates the outer shell of the egg, a chemical reaction prevents other sperm following suit. Twenty-three chromosomes from the sperm fuse with 23 chromosomes from the ovum to form a cell with 46 chromosomes (a zygote). This zygote repeatedly divides as it passes down the fallopian tube to form a ball of cells known as a morula. Fluid accumulates inside the morula to form a hollow bag of cells, and this implants itself in the receptive uterine lining approximately five days after fertilisation.

42. Is pre-conception preparation important?

The prospective mother and father should both consider improving their health prior to conceiving. Both should avoid smoking, alcohol, and all drugs if possible. Smoking and alcohol impair the quality of sperm, as does excessive ejaculation or prolonged abstinence. Sex every two to three days maintains semen at a volume in excess of 2 ml, with at least 20

PREGNANCY

million sperm per ml and with more than 60–75% normal, motile sperm.

The mother's diet is as important during the three months prior to pregnancy as during the pregnancy itself. Eat no more than 35% of daily calories as fat, with no more than 11% as saturated fat. Fat counters are available in newsagents to make calculation relatively simple. Increase your intake of protein and carbohydrate and take in adequate natural-source vitamins, minerals and fibre. Folic acid supplements were previously recommended just for women with a previous history of a child with a neural tube defect (such as spina bifida). Now, folate supplements of 0.4 mg per day are advised for *all* pregnant women to prevent a first occurrence of this unfortunate condition. As folate is important during the first month of gestation when the neural tube develops, taking them prior to conception may be a good idea. If you can't find a single vitamin supplement, buy one containing a B group complex with folic acid at a level of around 0.4 milligrams per day.

The obese should lose weight before becoming pregnant. Average weight gain during pregnancy is 12.5–14 kg (approximately two stone). Any more than this is excessive fat and will increase the likelihood of a large baby, diabetes of pregnancy, problems during labour and instrumental delivery (Caesarean section or forceps).

Pregnancy-associated osteoporosis (thinning bones) is increasingly recognised as being a problem and can even result in bone fracture. Before and during pregnancy, increase the calcium in your diet (an extra daily pint of milk, other dairy products, dark green vegetables, dried legumes, margarine, etc). Regular exercise also helps to protect against it. Those affected are advised not to breast-feed.

The potential mother should have a blood test to make sure she is immune to rubella (German measles). If she is not, vaccination is strongly advised *before* pregnancy occurs.

Previously, doctors advised coming off the pill for at least three months before conception, to allow the body's hormonal cycles to adjust. This is less popular now – fertility is maximal soon after stopping the oral contraceptive pill. It seems a shame to waste this period of hyperfertility, especially in 'career' women over the age of 30 trying for a first child. There is a trend for putting women on the pill prior to treatment for infertility – surprisingly, this increases their chance of pregnancy! There are cases where prolonged use of the pill can decrease fertility for up to a year. However, the pill does not cause long-term fertility problems.

43. *How can I tell if I'm pregnant?*

Fertilisation usually occurs in the middle of the menstrual cycle. By the time your period is one day overdue, you may already be two weeks pregnant! As the placenta develops, it secretes a hormone called human chorionic gonadotrophin (HCG) which is detectable in blood as early as 48 hours after conception, and in the urine 72 hours after conception. Pregnancy tests are remarkably accurate. Use a home kit or take a sample of early morning urine to a pharmacist.

The ovary secretes oestrogens and progesterone in high quantities and this accounts for the early

PREGNANCY

symptoms of pregnancy: nausea; tingling, tender breasts with distended superficial veins and darkening of the nipples; increased blood flow to the genitals resulting in a bluish tinge to the vagina and softening of the cervix. A doctor may detect this on examination, but internal examinations at this time are not popular. If a spontaneous miscarriage were to occur the woman might feel the examination was to blame.

44. *Why does miscarriage occur?*

It is estimated that 40–60% of all conceptions end in miscarriage, most before the mother is even aware that she was pregnant. The majority of miscarried foetuses are genetically malformed – which is not surprising given that up to 40% of sperm show abnormalities when viewed under the microscope, and that ova deteriorate with increasing maternal age.

Sadly, around 15% of recognised pregnancies miscarry before 12 weeks of pregnancy. Twice as many 'threaten' to abort with spotting and/or period-like pains.

Most spontaneous miscarriages are due to non-recurring causes and the prognosis is good in more than 95% of women. Recurrent 'abortion' is medically said to occur when three consecutive pregnancies end in spontaneous miscarriage. The incidence is low – approximately 0.2% of pregnancies.

The causes of recurrent miscarriage are many – structural or genetic abnormalities of the foetus, uterine or cervical abnormalities, and maternal illnesses. Immunological problems, with the mother

WHAT WORRIES WOMEN MOST

rejecting antigens from her husband, are increasingly thought to be at fault. Exciting research aimed at desensitising women against their husbands' antigens (using white blood cells extracted from the father and injected into the mother) is currently proving successful.

45. *What tests can ensure that my baby is normal?*

Antenatal care revolves around determining 'risk' factors in a pregnancy and monitoring foetal development. Listening to the foetal heart, counting foetal movements, and measuring expansion of the womb, are all simple tests of well-being. Ultrasound scanning allows direct examination of the foetus through the abdominal wall, or occasionally through the vagina. Most maternity units perform routine scans at 16–20 weeks of pregnancy. Scanning measures foetal length, girth and head diameter to assess age, locates the placenta, and diagnoses anatomical abnormalities such as spina bifida, cleft lip, cystic kidneys, abnormal brain structure, etc. Sex can sometimes be predicted, but not always reliably.

Some maternity units measure an embryonic protein called alpha-fetoprotein in maternal blood at 16–18 weeks – high levels are associated with certain abnormalities, for example spina bifida, water on the brain, Down's syndrome, faulty development.

Amniocentesis is a process whereby a fine needle is inserted through the mother's abdomen to collect a sample of amniotic fluid surrounding the foetus. This allows genetic examination of foetal cells and

PREGNANCY

detects genetic problems such as Down's syndrome. Research is currently looking at the causes of enzyme deficiencies leading to conditions such as cystic fibrosis.

Amniocentesis accurately determines the baby's gender, which proves useful in sex-linked conditions such as Duchenne's Dystrophy, a muscular disease which tends to affect boys. Amniocentesis does carry a small risk of miscarriage (0.5–1%) and cannot safely be performed prior to 16 weeks.

In chorionic villus sampling the placenta is tested for the same conditions as amniocentesis. A biopsy is made on small amounts of tissue from the placenta. This can be done as early as 8 weeks pregnancy but carries a 1–2% risk of miscarriage.

The latest technique involves viewing the foetus directly (from 5 weeks of pregnancy) via an endoscope passed through the cervic (embryoscopy). This picks up a range of genetic syndromes too subtle to be identified by ultrasound at such an early stage. The advantage of this procedure over tests performed later (at 16 weeks) is that if a therapeutic abortion is requested, termination is much less traumatic for all concerned. There is a small risk of miscarriage with embryoscopy – comparable to that of amniocentesis – of 0.5–1%. This technique provides an access route for future gene therapy. At present, the only human tissue that can be used for cell transfer into an embryo is bone marrow. Many ethical and legal considerations need to be addressed before the full potential of embryoscopy is realised.

WHAT WORRIES WOMEN MOST

46. Is it safe to take exercise during pregnancy?

It is safe to continue a regular exercise programme during pregnancy. There is no evidence to suggest that moderate exercise results in premature birth, even towards the end of term. Swimming and cycling are particularly good as they improve strength, stamina and suppleness without stressing weight-bearing joints. Avoid 'high-impact' sports such as sprinting, advanced aerobics and skiing, or activities such as horse-riding where falling is a possibility.

Towards the end of pregnancy, ligaments in the back and pelvis become slack due to the effects of progesterone and a hormone called relaxin. As a result, joint aches and pains can become a problem. The increasing bulk of breasts and abdomen will also naturally curtail your activities. The simple rule to follow is: if you feel uncomfortable or tired, *stop*.

47. What methods of pain relief are available during labour? Are they safe?

Antenatal preparation, resulting in an understanding of the process involved during labour, is consistently shown to reduce the need for pain-killing drugs. Similarly, the mother's confidence in the attending midwife lowers anxiety and the level at which pain is perceived.

Women vary in how they experience labour pains. Some claim to feel no pain and experience a floating,

PREGNANCY

euphoric state – possibly induced by their brain's own heroin-like chemicals. Nitrous oxide ('laughing gas') is a powerful and safe pain-killer if administered with 50% oxygen. Many women find breathing this enough to cope with peak contractions.

Pethidine, administered as an intramuscular injection every four hours, provides adequate pain relief but needs to be tailed off as delivery approaches. It has a sedative effect and may interfere with the baby's initial attempts at breathing.

Epidural anaesthesia is popular as it gives total pain relief. The mother remains fully conscious throughout, but pushing during delivery may be ineffective. Forceps extraction is therefore more likely. The administering of epidural injections is a skilled procedure which sometimes fails for technical reasons. If drugs are delivered into the wrong place, low blood pressure may result. A small, first test dose is designed to recognise and prevent this. Rarely, a toxic reaction to the local anaesthetic or an accidental overdose may be fatal. Some women seem to suffer chronic back pains, pins and needles or numbness following epidural injection.

Perhaps the safest form of analgesia during labour is acupuncture. Used by a skilled practitioner on a receptive patient, it significantly raises pain thresholds and is now available in many maternity units.

Stimulating nerves at the base of the spine with electrical impulses blocks the conduction of pain messages in the dorsal columns of the spinal cord and gives relief to many women. It is totally safe

WHAT WORRIES WOMEN MOST

and is known as TENS (transcutaneous electrical nerve stimulation).

48. Will I need an episiotomy?

An episiotomy is a controlled cut made from the vagina, through the perineum, and usually to one side of the anus. It was once universally practised on all women having their first baby. Now, it is performed less often – in 35% of all deliveries but well over 50% of first births.

Most obstetricians agree that episiotomy should only be used if specifically advisable. When the possible alternative of a third degree tear is considered (the vagina splitting into the rectum), episiotomy is viewed in better perspective. An episiotomy is easier to repair and usually heals better than a tear.

Many women worry about episiotomy. By the time the cut is made, vaginal and perineal tissues are already stretched paper-thin. There is usually time to administer a local anaesthetic first. If timed correctly, when crowning of the foetal head is imminent, episiotomy leads to delivery of the head. Care is taken that delivery is not too quick, or further tearing and extension of the cut are possible.

Time and skill are essential commodities during episiotomy repair. Poor needlework can result in chronic discomfort and problems when making love.

If you have reservations about episiotomy, talk these over with your doctor and midwife prior to delivery.

PREGNANCY

49. Is breast milk better than the bottle?

Breast-feeding has undeniably reduced disease and mortality in the Third World but for some reason it is often shunned in developed countries although recommended by doctors. Medically, it is the best option for any infant. Breast milk confers immunity against childhood disease and reduces the incidence of infection. Babies exclusively breast-fed up to 13 weeks of age are four times less likely to get gastro-intestinal symptoms such as vomiting and diarrhoea.

Premature babies fed on breast milk are 20 times less likely to develop the severe bowel disease 'necrotising enterocolitis', which has a 25% death rate, than babies fed on bottled milk formulae. Breast-feeding reduces the severity of infantile eczema and may increase IQ, especially in premature babies, as nutritionally it is complete.

Recent studies in Australia and New Zealand suggest that breast-fed babies are less likely to suffer cot death syndrome. This has prompted both governments to recommend breast-feeding as a specific strategy in reducing the risk of sudden infant death.

Breast-feeding is so beneficial to a child that, despite the fact that the HIV virus can be passed on in milk, the World Health Organisation have urged all women to continue breast-feeding. They state: 'A child's risk of dying of AIDS through breast-feeding must be balanced against its risk of dying of other causes if not breast-fed.' Studies in Africa and

WHAT WORRIES WOMEN MOST

Europe show the vast majority of babies breast-fed by HIV-positive mothers do not become infected.

In the UK, 65% of mothers breast-feed their newborn babies, but only 26% of babies are still breast-fed by the age of four months. Social class and education are important factors. Latest figures show that 79% of mothers in non-manual worker groups choose to breast-feed their babies compared to 57% in manual worker groups.

Ninety-three per cent of mothers who remained in full-time education until the age of 19 choose breast-feeding rather than the bottle, compared to 57% of first-time mothers who left school at 16 years.

Some women who want to breast-feed find they are not able to. Sometimes they do not produce enough milk, or their nipples become very sore. These problems often disappear within a few days, so it may be worth persisting for a while. Another difficulty is inverted nipples. A suction device to pull out the nipples has recently been developed.

CYSTITIS

Cystitis is an inflammation or infection of the bladder. Fifty per cent of women will suffer it at least once during their life. Experience symptoms include burning when passing urine, a frequent need to go to the toilet – often to pass tiny amounts – and a sense of urgency to empty the bladder before losing control. Backache and fever may occur, with the urine smelling unpleasant and looking cloudy or stained with fresh blood.

50. Why do I keep getting cystitis?

Cystitis seems to plague some women while others never suffer at all. Anatomy is partly to blame: the urethra (the tube from the bladder to the outside) is much shorter in women than in men, and bacteria therefore ascend more easily to cause infection.

Recurrent cystitis may be triggered by bacteria pushed into the urethra during frequent sexual intercourse ('honeymoon cystitis'). This is more likely the closer the urethra and vagina are physically sited. In some women the urethra opens just below the clitoris, while in others it opens into the lower vagina.

Some infections result from wiping the bottom from back to front or poor technique during insertion of tampons. Cystitis regularly occurs after practices such as anal sex, anal fingering during intercourse, and oral sex (cunnilingus) unless hygiene is rigorously attended to. Even wearing tight trousers has been known to initiate an attack.

WHAT WORRIES WOMEN MOST

Detergents and perfumes often cause chemical inflammation of the urethra (urethritis) and upset the acid and bacterial balance of the female genitalia. This lowers local resistance to infection and encourages conditions such as cystitis and thrush. Some sexually transmissible diseases (herpes, chlamydia, trichomonas) also invade the urethra and can cause classic recurrent symptoms of cystitis.

Progesterone has a relaxant effect on smooth muscle. Cystitis is therefore more common during the second half of the menstrual cycle, during pregnancy, and while on the pill. Conditions which can cause recurrent cystitis are diabetes, anaemia, and anatomical abnormalities of the urinary system. Cystitis can occasionally ascend to infect the kidneys, resulting in the more serious condition of pyelonephritis.

51. What self-help remedies are available for cystitis?

As soon as you display symptoms of cystitis, drink a pint of water. Then drink half a pint every 20 minutes if you can. Fluids help flush the urinary system through and may be enough to cure the problem. You'll soon start going to the loo regularly. Urination may sting initially but will improve as you continue to empty your bladder. It is best to drink water, but milk, weak tea or other bland substances will do. Avoid acidic liquids such as cola or fruit juice. These will irritate inflamed tissues more.

Unless you suffer from high blood pressure or heart trouble, drink a teaspoon of bicarbonate of

CYSTITIS

soda mixed with water every hour for three hours. This makes the urine less acid and relieves discomfort, as well as discouraging multiplication of bacteria.

Simple remedies such as paracetamol, a hot-water bottle and resting with your feet up will help. After three hours of this regime, symptoms should start to improve. If symptoms last longer than a day, if you are pregnant or if there is obvious blood in your urine, consult your doctor as soon as possible. A urine test and antibiotics may be prescribed. Cystitis in men or children should always be referred to a doctor.

For prevention of recurrent cystitis, hygiene is all-important. Wash with warm, unperfumed soapy water after every bowel movement and after sex. When sitting on the toilet, tilt your pelvis so the anus is lower than the urethra. After emptying the bowels or urinating, and while still on the toilet with your pelvis tilted, try using a bottle to pour warm soapy water between your legs and down the perineum between the vulva and the anus. This rapidly washes material from the bowels away from the urethra. If cystitis continues to plague your life, local application of an antiseptic cream such as cetrimide may help.

Always drink more than three pints of fluid per day.

Many women have found their chronic cystitis cured with homeopathic remedies.

STRESS INCONTINENCE

According to a recent MORI poll, at least 3½ million people in Britain suffer from urinary incontinence – and possibly as many as 10 million.

Some studies suggest that 60% of menopausal women experience leakage of urine, though it is not just confined to this age group. One in ten women aged 15 to 64 admit to wetting themselves at least twice a month!

Some cases of incontinence are mild, with only slight damping when coughing or sneezing occurs. Other victims are devastated by a total loss of bladder control. Half of all sufferers never consult their doctor, because of either embarrassment or a mistaken belief that 'nothing can be done'. What is not appreciated is that seven out of ten cases of incontinence are curable.

The commonest form of incontinence in women is stress incontinence.

52. What causes stress incontinence?

'Stress' incontinence refers to a physical and not a psychological problem. Weakness of the pelvic floor muscles is at fault, resulting in sagging of the bladder neck, and sometimes the vaginal walls or uterus prolapse (see Question 61).

Lack of oestrogen after the menopause plays a part, but almost invariably, weakness of the pelvic floor results from difficult or repeated childbirth.

Lack of pelvic floor support places strain on muscles that keep the bladder and urethral openings

STRESS INCONTINENCE

closed. A sudden increase in pressure as happens during lifting, coughing, laughing, sneezing or running then results in urine leaking out.

Many sufferers cut down on their fluid intake in an attempt to 'dry' things up. In fact, this usually makes things worse. Urine becomes concentrated, more irritant, and is more likely to produce a detectable smell. As with cystitis, it's important to maintain an adequate fluid intake of at least three litres a day.

53. What can be done for stress incontinence?

Initially it is important to send a urine sample to the hospital to exclude infection which may compound the problem. Your doctor will then gently examine you to assess your pelvic organs and look for any prolapse. There are no satisfactory drugs available to treat stress incontinence. The best approach is physiotherapy to increase pelvic floor muscle tone or surgical suspension of the bladder neck.

A continence adviser will suggest exercises to help you. A simple one is to pull up the front and back passages tightly as if trying to stop the bowels from opening. Hold tight for a count of four and repeat this every quarter of an hour.

When on the loo, practise stopping the flow of urine mid-stream. Initially this will be difficult, but when it becomes easy, do this at least once a day for improvement. Pull in the pelvic floor muscles before coughing, sneezing or lifting, and avoid

What Worries Women Most

standing for long periods of time. Often, these simple measures result in dramatic improvement.

Physiotherapists can electrically stimulate the pelvic floor and provide weighted cones for insertion, which tighten and tone vaginal muscles.

Surgery has a 95% success rate and involves stitching a nylon 'sling' under the neck of the bladder to provide support. Tucks are usually taken into the vaginal walls to simultaneously tighten them and as a bonus, many women find this also improves their sex life.

Prolapse of the uterus may contribute to stress incontinence and if your family is complete, a vaginal hysterectomy may be the best option. This can be performed at the same time as surgery to support the bladder neck and has the advantage of not leaving an abdominal scar.

THRUSH

Thrush is caused by *Candida albicans*, a microscopic, yeast-like fungus. Seventy-five per cent of women will experience vaginal thrush at least once in their life, but some are plagued with never-ending recurrences.

54. What are the symptoms of genital thrush?

Thrush infection can sometimes be 'silent', with spores (reproductive bodies) present but quiescent in a so-called 'carrier' state. When activated, threads of fungal material (hyphae) burrow between vaginal lining cells to cause fissures and the common symptoms of itching, soreness, pain on intercourse, dryness and a white, cottage-cheese-like discharge. This smells pleasantly like commercial yeast extract.

In severe cases, vaginal tissues become swollen and glands in the groin enlarge. The whole area is very tender and passing urine may be painful. The vagina can be packed full of thick, white curds but sometimes only a few white plaques are visible on the vaginal walls. The quantity of discharge does not necessarily equate with severity of symptoms.

On the penis, thrush looks like small red spots on the 'helmet'. There may also be soreness and a build-up of white material under the foreskin.

55. Why do I get recurrent thrush?

Thrush spores are present in the air and germinate in warm, moist places. Candida thrives when natural immunity falls during times of stress and illness.

WHAT WORRIES WOMEN MOST

Antibiotic therapy kills bacteria which normally colonise the healthy gut and vagina. This removes ecosystem competition and provides a niche for Candida to thrive.

High oestrogen levels occurring while on the pill, during pregnancy, and in the second half of the menstrual cycle increase the glycogen (sugar) content of vaginal cells. Together with falling acidity of secretions which also occurs at these times, conditions are ripe for thrush.

Recurrent thrush may be associated with iron-deficiency anaemia, low blood levels of the iron-carrying protein ferritin, and diabetes, all of which your GP will screen you for.

Trauma to vaginal tissues from vigorous sex, or even rubbing too hard with a bath towel, allows thrush to penetrate.

If you're being treated for Candida, make sure your partner uses an anti-thrush cream too. Thrush spores can survive under the male foreskin without causing problems. They may then be passed back to you.

56. What thrush treatments are available?

Creams for application to the skin and pre-filled syringes of vaginal preparations can now be bought from pharmacists. Your GP can prescribe pessaries and tampons impregnated with anti-thrush drugs if you prefer.

For recurrent thrush, oral courses (varying from one to four tablets) can eradicate reservoirs of Candida infection in the gut. Many women have

THRUSH

found relief from thrush with homeopathic treatments. Self-help remedies include:

- smearing the vulval area with yoghurt containing a live culture of *Lactobacillus acidophilus*. This will colonise the vagina and oust thrush invaders. Check the label of your yoghurt for this particular culture before buying – it's the only culture that will work. It can usually be found in health food shops;
- not using bath additives, vaginal deodorants or douches. All destroy the protective acid mantle of the vagina;
- wearing loose clothing with cotton gussets. Tights, nylon panties and close-fitting trousers increase warmth and humidity in the groin;
- hot-ironing pantie gussets. Modern low-temperature washing-machine cycles don't always kill Candida spores.

VAGINAL DISCHARGE

The vagina is the most efficient self-cleansing organ in the body. Despite this, discharges commonly worry women – either because they're too copious or because they have an unpleasant smell.

Sending a vaginal swab to hospital for culture and microscopy often proves unhelpful. Few bugs survive well enough to be detected and infection is frequently missed. If you suspect discharge problems it is best to attend a genito-urinary (sometimes known as VD, STD, or Special) clinic where fresh microscopy is performed. In addition, a special cervical swab will be taken for detection of Chlamydia (see Question 57).

When viewed under the microscope, healthy vaginal discharge consists mainly of bacteria, dead vaginal lining cells, mucus, and often a smattering of sperm. When infection is present, pus cells give a greenish-yellow tinge to secretions, and disease-causing organisms may be identified.

The best bacteria for colonising your vagina are *Lactobacillus acidophilus* – a bug equally at home in up-market un-pasteurised yoghurt.

Most bacteria in the vagina are 'aerobic' – meaning not that they regularly exercise but that they need oxygen to survive. A minority of vaginal bacterial are 'anaerobic' and prefer a low oxygen saturation. Bacterial imbalances do occur when anaerobes over-grow and oust protective lactobacilli. This causes an increased, smelly discharge often accompanied by soreness. Only a few antibiotics are able to redress this imbalance – metronidazole

VAGINAL DISCHARGE

(which frequently causes nausea and is poisonous in combination with alcohol) and co-amoxyclav (a souped-up version of penicillin).

57. *What causes excess vaginal discharge?*

A famous gynaecologist (male) once stated that if a woman didn't have a vaginal discharge, she'd start to squeak as she walked.

In the majority of women complaining of excess vaginal discharge, no condition needing treatment can be found. It is then said to be 'physiological' (a normal function of the body). Certain high-oestrogen states, such as pregnancy or the oral contraceptive pill, encourage physiological vaginal discharge – often because a cervical 'erosion' is present. This results when endocervical cells, normally found lining the cervical canal, grow over and replace the cells protecting the cervix on the vaginal side. Endocervical cells produce mucus. Therefore when an erosion is present, the number of mucus-secreting cells, and the quantity of physiological discharge, increase.

If you are on a contraceptive pill which is predominantly progestogenic, the opposite problem – vaginal dryness – can result. It's therefore often worth changing the pill to several different blends before assuming your discharge has to be lived with.

Gynaecological infections such as thrush (a yeast), trichomonas (a protozoan), Gardnerella (a bacterium) and anaerobic vaginosis (bacterial imbalance) can produce a discharge. These are usually suspected due to itch, soreness or smell. Primary herpes (the initial infection) produces copious watery secretions but is invariably intensely painful. Secondary herpetic recurrences sometimes only involve the cervix and may not be uncomfortable. In this case, increased watery discharge may be the only symptom noticed. Many women have found relief from herpes in homeopathic remedies.

It's always worth having increased vaginal discharge investigated, if only to exclude chlamydia (NSU). This is a sexually transmissible disease which, if untreated, can result in pelvic inflammation and sub-fertility. Unfortunately, it is often present without symptoms and may only be diagnosed by chance. Chlamydia are too small to be seen under an ordinary microscope and are extremely difficult to grow in the laboratory. They are detected in a cervical swab via an immunological technique which takes several days. If this infection is suspected, you will be treated with antibiotics before the result is through. It's better to treat if you haven't got it, than not to treat if you have.

Occasionally, on careful questioning, it becomes apparent that a complaint of excessive discharge coincides with stopping the use of condoms as a method of contraception!

58. Why do vaginal discharges smell?

Vaginal discharge has a number of distinct functions:

- it protects vaginal lining cells from drying out;
- it prevents chafing;
- it flushes the vagina clean;
- it provides lubrication during intercourse;

VAGINAL DISCHARGE

- it protects against infection;
- it acts as a sexual attractant to the male.

The last two functions are partly responsible for the characteristic female smell. One of the ways vaginal discharge protects against infection is through colonisation with healthy bacteria. These have metabolic pathways and excretion products of their own which contribute to odour.

Super-infection with agents causing disease (pathogens) changes vaginal odours from a fresh, slightly sweet smell with 'green' top-notes to sometimes rank, cheesy and unfortunately, frankly fishy, undertones. The worst offenders are anaerobes such as Gardnerella and Bacteroides. Candida (thrush) imparts a pleasant, slightly acidic odour reminiscent of yeast extracts. In some women, yeasts live quite happily in the vagina to contribute to odour and cause no obvious problems. They show up on routine smears and then tend to be eradicated with treatment.

The skin surrounding the vagina and anus contains special sweat glands which are also present in the armpit. These secrete small quantities of oily fluid said to be odourless on reaching the skin surface. Thereafter secretions develop a characteristic odour due to bacterial decomposition. These apocrine glands are derived from primitive organs similar to those in musk deer, the skunk and other lower mammals. The glands are responsible for territorial marking, species recognition and sexual attractants. Their secretions contain pheromones – chemicals finely tuned by evolution to sexually attract the opposite sex. There is no reason why our pubic apocrine glands should be any different. It's possible that if we didn't have such a characteristic vaginal odour, the human race would have died out many millennia ago! (see Question 15)

HYSTERECTOMY/PROBLEMS THAT CAN LEAD TO HYSTERECTOMY

Hysterectomy is the surgical removal of the womb. This may also include the removal of the ovaries and fallopian tubes and is one of the most emotive operations a woman can have. Around 66,000 are performed in England and Wales each year, but this number will soon fall. New techniques have been perfected which provide alternative treatment for several gynaecological disorders (see Question 67).

The womb is a pear-shaped, hollow muscle lying in the middle of the pelvis. Its bottom end (the cervix) communicates with the vagina and its top end with the ovaries via the fallopian tubes. Everything is held in place by a number of loose ligaments – rather like elastic bands.

Where possible, hysterectomy is performed vaginally as this is safer and avoids an abdominal scar.

59. *Do I need a hysterectomy?*

Women frequently consult their doctor with heavy, painful, irregular periods. These have a number of causes (see under 'Periods'). Some can be solved with tablets, but six conditions often result in the need for hysterectomy: fibroids, menorrhagia, prolapse, pelvic inflammatory disease, endometriosis (see below for all these) and gynaecological cancers. In the case of the last, hysterectomy is mandatory. Otherwise, hysterectomy is resorted to if a woman's quality of life is seriously affected by pain, heavy bleeding or exhaustion.

It is estimated that one in five women will need a hysterectomy by the time they reach 75. Women under the age of 30 who have been sterilised have three to four times the average chance of a hysterectomy in later years. There are two possible reasons:

- sterilisation may increase the risk of uterine disease;
- surgeons may be less reluctant to remove the womb in a woman who has already declared her family to be complete.

Occasionally, a woman seems keen to have a hysterectomy as a form of sterilisation, rather than because her periods are totally unbearable.

60. What are fibroids?

Fibroids are benign tumours of uterine muscle. Up to a third of women get them, especially if they've had several pregnancies. Fibroids can also prove hereditary.

Fibroids prevent the ordered contraction of uterine muscle and expand the surface area of the lining of the womb. This results in prolonged, heavy, painful periods (menorrhagia). In extreme cases, fibroids can enlarge the womb by as much as a 20-week foetus!

Fibroids can be 'shelled out' with a giant corkscrew but if no further pregnancies are required, a hysterectomy may be recommended – especially if blood loss is heavy enough to induce anaemia. Occasionally, fibroids result in life-threatening haemorrhage and hysterectomy becomes an emergency, life-saving procedure.

HYSTERECTOMY

61. What is a prolapse?

When muscles and ligaments supporting the female organs stretch, prolapse may occur. Horror stories of the bottom falling out of your world (and vice versa) are only slightly accurate. In very few cases does the womb actually drop outside the body. Usually it stays half-way down the vagina but may poke out on straining down. Gently insert a finger an inch into your vagina and bear downwards as though trying to open your bowels. If you feel a firm, rubbery cone (the cervix) rushing towards you there may be a degree of prolapse.

Sometimes the bladder bulges backwards into the vagina or the rectum bulges forwards. This may be accompanied by 'stress incontinence' (see Question 52).

Stretching of ligaments is due to bearing large babies and to difficult and prolonged labour. Symptoms may not arise until after the menopause, when ligaments thin (atrophy) due to lack of oestrogen.

Prolapses are uncomfortable, interfere with your sex life, and can cause problems when passing water or defecating. A few also result in unpleasant sensations of 'something coming down'. If you suspect you may have a degree of prolapse, consult your doctor who will examine you internally and assess what treatment is necessary. If surgical repair is recommended, vaginal hysterectomy is often performed at the same time.

62. What is endometriosis?

Cells usually found in the lining of the womb (endometrium) sometimes exist elsewhere in the body. It's thought that backward bleeding during a period forces cells into the abdominal cavity via the fallopian tubes. Rarely, endometrial cells enter the blood supply and travel to other organs such as the lungs.

These displaced endometrial cells still respond to hormonal cycles and bleed into surrounding tissues during menstruation. 'Chocolate' cysts filled with decaying blood may form in pockets of endometriosis peppering the outside surfaces of pelvic organs. A build-up of inflammation and scarring then occurs. Structures such as the bowel and bladder mat together and intense, chronic pain develops. Intercourse is often impossible.

Hormonal manipulation (for example with the pill) is tried as a first-line treatment. Keyhole surgery to cut away adhesions, and diathermy (burning out) of small areas and cysts, may help. In severe cases, hysterectomy and pelvic clearance (which includes ovaries, fallopian tubes and scar tissue) may be the only option.

63. What is pelvic inflammatory disease?

Pelvic Inflammatory Disease (PID) results from an ascending infection of the female genital tract. Eighty per cent of cases are caused by sexually transmissible diseases (for example chlamydia or gonorrhoea) plus anaerobic bacteria. Infection may

HYSTERECTOMY

also ascend after termination of pregnancy or implantation of a coil. It is estimated that 15% of all women born between 1945 and 1954 have had PID by the age of 30.

After one attack of PID, 80% of sufferers will experience heavy or irregular periods and 40% will suffer deep pain during sexual intercourse. Twenty per cent of sufferers will experience chronic pelvic pain and 13% will become infertile. The risk of ectopic pregnancy (implantation of a fertilised egg somewhere other than the womb, for example in the fallopian tube) is seven times greater in women who have experienced PID.

After a second attack of PID, infertility rates rise to 35%. After a third episode, 75% of women are infertile – due to scarring and blockage of the fallopian tubes.

PID starts as infection of the endometrium, fallopian tubes and ovaries and may extend beyond the pelvis to inflame the appendix, peritoneum and even the surface of the liver.

Unfortunately, inflammation and scarring results in poor penetration of antibiotics into the fallopian tubes where infection lurks. Treatment therefore consists of at least 14 days' therapy with two or even three different antibiotics. Sometimes, admission to hospital for antibiotic injections is necessary. Sexual partners should *always* be examined to prevent re-infection of the woman once she has recovered and resumes an active sex life.

If the pain from subsequent inflammation or adhesions (bands of internal scar tissue) is excessive, sexual intercourse becomes impossible. Sometimes even walking proves difficult. Hysterectomy may then become a last resort.

WHAT WORRIES WOMEN MOST

64. What happens during hysterectomy?

Hysterectomy only occurs with the informed consent of the woman involved. It should never be forced upon you. Together, you and your gynaecologist will decide whether vaginal or abdominal hysterectomy is preferable. Vaginal operation has the advantage of no abdominal scar and recovery is usually sooner. The vagina may require tightening and if you have problems with stress incontinence, the bladder neck can be supported at the same time.

Until recently, vaginal hysterectomy was unavailable to women suffering adhesions or those also requiring removal of diseased ovaries. The latest technique, 'laparoscopically assisted vaginal hysterectomy', uses a viewing device (laparoscope) and surgical instruments which are inserted through three tiny scars on the abdominal wall. After gas is pumped in to improve access, adhesions are finely divided. The abdomen is then deflated and the hysterectomy completed vaginally. Another advantage of this technique is that no internal stitching is involved – an adapted stapling technique is used and women are able to return to work in a very short time.

During abdominal hysterectomy, a bikini-line scar is preferred. If you have large fibroids or a significant ovarian cyst, a vertical scar may be necessary for easier access.

Originally, sub-total hysterectomy was performed which left the cervix in place. Now, total hysterectomy is preferred as removing the cervix prevents future development of cervical cancer.

HYSTERECTOMY

Wertheim's hysterectomy is used when treating cancer. It involves cutting away the upper vagina, ligaments, lymph glands and fatty tissues, and is also known as pelvic clearance.

65. Will I lose my ovaries when having a hysterectomy?

In younger women, the ovaries are retained where possible to prevent an early menopause. If the ovaries are diseased (cysts, endometriosis) or if you are approaching the menopause, removal of the womb, fallopian tubes and ovaries *en masse* may be recommended. This guards against subsequent ovarian cancer. Hormone Replacement Therapy will be prescribed six weeks after the operation, often as an abdominal wall implant.

Interestingly, when ovaries are left in place, 25% of women experience the menopause within two years. It is thought there is an as-yet unrecognised interaction between the ovaries and the uterus, causing ovaries to fail after a hysterectomy.

66. Will I be less feminine or lose my sex drive after a hysterectomy?

Psychological problems, including depression and feelings of lost femininity, may occur after hysterectomy. Proper counselling before and after the operation helps minimise this. If a woman reaches her own decision about the necessity for a hysterectomy, few emotional problems tend to occur. Often, a woman is so grateful for the cessation of pain,

WHAT WORRIES WOMEN MOST

menorrhagia or Pre-Menstrual Syndrome that the operation transforms her life.

Sudden withdrawal of oestrogen if the ovaries are removed can cause depression as part of the menopause symptom complex. Once HRT is commenced six weeks after the operation, this will improve.

Sexual intercourse can resume six weeks after hysterectomy. Take your time and ensure adequate lubrication with K-Y jelly or pessaries. Orgasm may, however, feel 'different'. A study in Japan found that 27% of hysterectomised women experienced loss of uterine sensation while making love, and 70% claimed difficulty in reaching an orgasm.

A similar survey in Finland compared women who had had a total hysterectomy with those who had had a partial hysterectomy (this leaves the cervix and vagina intact). Researchers found no difference in sexual desire between the two groups but after one year, there was a significant reduction in frequency of orgasm amongst the women who had undergone a total hysterectomy.

Deep muscular contractions during orgasm will no longer involve the uterus and attached ligaments after hysterectomy. Some women, however, find this intensifies clitoral sensations and claim their enjoyment of clitoral orgasm has vastly improved.

67. *What are the alternatives to hysterectomy?*

Lasers and tiny cutting tools are starting to take over from the surgeon's knife. Traditional indications for hysterectomy such as heavy bleeding (menorrhagia)

HYSTERECTOMY

and painful periods (dysmenorrhoea) can be dealt with by minimally invasive endoscopic (keyhole) techniques.

Endometrial removal (ablation) involves a course of tablets (danazol) to thin down the lining of the womb. A laser is then inserted into the uterus and dragged over the endometrium to vaporise the tissue. Endometrial resection is similar except that an endoscopic cutting tool is used to pare away the endometrium, down as far as uterine muscle.

Both procedures result in either no periods or acceptably light ones. The operations take 20 minutes and can be done on a day-case basis under general or local anaesthesia.

Fifty per cent of women undergoing hysterectomy are eligible for ablation or resection instead. This could save the NHS up to £50 million per year!

Another technique uses microwaves to destroy the endometrium. The 'Menostat' is currently undergoing clinical trials. This has an intra-uterine probe designed to reach the corners of the womb, and generates a heat gradient to kill endometrial cells. Guards in the vagina and rectum prevent unwanted damage to other tissues.

MENOPAUSE

Medical diagnosis of the menopause is only made 'retrospectively' after a woman has experienced no periods for a year. The average age at which it occurs is 51. As most modern women live into their 80s, 40% of our active lives may be considered post-menopausal! Many women find they start the menopause at the same age as their mothers.

Interestingly, smoking cigarettes brings the menopause on 1–2 years earlier (by increasing processing of oestrogen and reducing blood levels). There is evidence that passive smoking hastens events too.

If the menopause occurs before the age of 44, it is premature and a result of ovarian failure.

The climacteric (or 'change of life') represents the transition from fertility to infertility. Twenty-five per cent of women have no symptoms at all, 50% experience mild symptoms associated with hormone withdrawal, but another 25% will suffer symptoms so severely they may feel life isn't worth living.

The main symptoms experienced during the menopause are: hot flushes (75% of women); night sweats (40%); tiredness (40%); irritability (30%); unstable emotions (30%); insomnia (30%); and depression (30%). Vaginal discomfort and urinary problems may also affect some women.

A woman who has had a hysterectomy will go through the menopause five years earlier on average than other women, even when the ovaries are left intact.

MENOPAUSE

68. Will my sex drive dwindle after the menopause?

Women's experiences vary greatly. Interest in sex is as much to do with mental attitude and physical fitness as hormonal changes. Some women find their libido is lowered because they feel tired, depressed and sweaty. Others find their interest in sex increases – possibly due to the increased influence of the hormone testosterone in a lowered oestrogen environment.

Most studies do show a decline in the frequency of sexual activity after the menopause. This may be due to declining sexual capacity in the male and the increased prevalence of erectile failure with age (35% of over-60s). A recent survey in the USA found that amongst people aged 60 years and over, 56% of married women and 5% of unmarried women were still sexually active. More men claimed to be sexually active than women.

Vaginal dryness can be a problem after the menopause. Secretion of vaginal lubrication is an oestrogen-dependent process, but this is easily overcome with K-Y lubricating pessaries or jelly.

With thinning of tissues that occurs in the absence of oestrogen, the clitoris may become less sensitive, or even unpleasantly hypersensitive. Longer foreplay may be required to reach orgasm. With an understanding partner, your sex life shouldn't take a dive through what can be a difficult time. Hormone Replacement Therapy (HRT) will offset most symptoms, including low libido.

WHAT WORRIES WOMEN MOST

As post-menopausal years advance, oestrogen deficiency causes shortening and narrowing of the vagina and shrinkage of the opening. Cushioning tissues (fat, collagen) around the vagina atrophy, and the piston-like action of sex may be uncomfortable. Experimenting with different coital positions (use a manual if necessary) should help you to find an acceptable compromise.

69. *What are the risks and benefits of hormone replacement therapy?*

It is important to realise that HRT and the contraceptive pill are very different. HRT restores oestrogen levels to the 'low normal' range in women experiencing ovarian failure. The total monthly dose taken is much less than would be secreted by the ovaries in a normal menstrual cycle. The contraceptive pill, on the other hand, deliberately increases hormone levels above normal to approximate those of pregnancy. These high doses suppress ovarian activity.

The type of oestrogen used in the pill is usually synthetic, while HRT tends to contain natural oestrogens. For both the above reasons, the risks and benefits of HRT are different from those of the pill.

Studies show that HRT reduces the risk of coronary heart disease in women past the menopause by up to 50%. In women who have already had a heart attack, HRT provides 80% protection against another one occurring. As a 50-year-old woman not on HRT has a 46% chance of developing coronary

MENOPAUSE

heart disease and a 31% chance of dying from it, the protection given by HRT is significant.

Oestrogen has this effect by lowering blood cholesterol (LDLs – see Question 93), by preserving arterial wall elasticity and by discouraging atherosclerosis (hardening and furring up of the arteries).

A 50-year-old woman has a 20% chance of suffering a stroke during the rest of her life and an 8% chance of dying from one. Some studies show HRT has a beneficial effect on these figures, others don't. Overall, the effect of HRT on strokes is probably neutral.

Perhaps the most worrying association with HRT is the risk of developing breast cancer. A 50-year-old woman not on HRT has a 10% risk of developing breast cancer during the rest of her life and a 3% chance of dying from it. Studies suggest that using HRT for more than eight years increases the risk of breast cancer to 12½%.

However, women using HRT *before* developing breast cancer may actualy have a lower risk of *death* from breast cancer than those *not* taking HRT – because if they have used HRT and then develop breast cancer, subsequently stopping the HRT causes an oestrogen-dependent tumour to shrink.

Overall, there is no evidence that oestrogen therapy substantially increases the risk of *dying* from breast cancer. One in 11 women will develop this disease anyway, whether or not they have had HRT. Best medical advice at present is that using HRT for five years will provide maximum benefit against heart disease and minimum risk of causing breast cancer.

WHAT WORRIES WOMEN MOST

A 50-year-old woman has a 50% chance of sustaining an osteoporotic bone fracture during the rest of her life and a 3% chance of dying as a result:

- a 15% risk of hip fracture;
- a 16% risk of wrist fracture;
- a 20–30% risk of spinal deformity from vertebral collapse.

Oestrogen slows bone loss and reduces the risk of developing a hip fracture by up to 40%. Bone loss continues once oestrogen therapy stops, and one study indicates protection against fractures is lost within five years of coming off HRT.

HRT users have half the risk of death from accidents, suicide and murder according to one survey – which may indicate a beneficial effect on emotions and personal interactions!

As long as non-hysterectomised women are prescribed cycles of progestogens with their oestrogen replacement therapy, the risk of developing womb cancer is not increased. Unopposed oestrogen causes over-growth of the womb lining and increases the risk of endometrial cancer by a factor of eight.

Taking all risks and benefits of HRT into account, the life expectancy of a 50-year-old woman taking combined oestrogen/progestogen HRT is expected to rise by almost a year according to computer simulations. However, women who already have an increased risk of breast cancer (that is, one or two direct relatives with the disease) gain little or no increase in life expectancy from HRT.

Taking HRT for five years minimises the risk of developing breast cancer and strongly protects against heart attack. It also 'buys' the skeleton five

MENOPAUSE

crucial years against osteoporosis and improves quality of life by controlling menopausal symptoms.

Decisions about taking HRT involve individual subjective judgments. Some women regard the small increased risk of breast cancer as more important than the large reduction in risk of heart disease – especially if a friend or relative has suffered. Other women may want, above all, to prevent hip fracture or osteoporotic wedge fractures of the vertebrae resulting in spinal deformity.

The severity of menopausal symptoms is certainly controlled by using HRT and some women opt to take HRT for six to 12 months to see them through this difficult period.

Possible side-effects of HRT include: breast tenderness; leg cramps; headache; nausea; water retention; rashes; jaundice (rarely); and withdrawal bleeds. Many of these disappear after three months' therapy and HRT should not be stopped without consultation with your prescribing physician.

Women not suited to HRT include those with: active blood or clotting disorders; strokes or transient ischaemic attacks (TIAs – tiny strokes lasting less than 24 hours); deteriorating hearing (due to otosclerosis); liver problems; fibroids and oestrogen-dependent tumours; and undiagnosed vaginal bleeding.

Doctors will not usually prescribe HRT to women with a previous history of breast cancer, but many specialists now feel this is not an absolute no-no.

WHAT WORRIES WOMEN MOST

70. Can I have the HRT patch?

Yes, as long as you are eligible for HRT. Until recently, hormone replacement patches only contained oestrogen. A delivery system through the skin has now been perfected for progesterone and patches for combined therapy are available.

Patches are stuck on the bottom or abdomen and changed twice a week. Those with an intact uterus require cyclical progestogen (either tablets or the combined patch) for 12 days in each cycle to prevent over-stimulation of the endometrium. This can lead to a pre-cancerous condition known as cystic hyperplasia. This is diagnosed via an endometrial biopsy and microscopic examination of tissue. Cyclical progesterone prevents cystic hyperplasia by inducing monthly shedding of the endometrium.

71. Will HRT mean my periods return?

If you haven't had a hysterectomy, most combined preparations of HRT will cause regular vaginal bleeding. This is usually light, and necessary to prevent over-stimulation of the endometrium (see Question 70).

One brand of HRT differs from the rest. It contains a single synthetic hormone called tibolone which possesses both oestrogenic and progestogenic properties. It is taken continuously, every day, and if prescribed to post-menopausal women who have not had a period for at least one year, there is unlikely to be a withdrawal bleed.

Because of its mode of action, tibolone does not

MENOPAUSE

overstimulate the endometrium and is not associated with cystic hyperplasia.

Trials are currently looking at taking certain blends of HRT continuously so that withdrawal bleeding doesn't occur.

72. What is the significance of post-menopausal bleeding?

Vaginal bleeding appearing more than six months after you thought your periods had stopped should be thought of as 'post-menopausal bleeding' (PMB), and a medical opinion sought without delay.

Bleeding occurring more than 12 months after the menopause needs investigation as a matter of urgency – even if it's only spotting.

In the majority of cases no cause is found – despite full investigation. Most diagnoses are non-serious but in 1% of single bleeds and 10% of recurrent PMBs a malignancy is discovered.

One of the commonest causes of PMB is a doctor prescribing HRT and forgetting to warn that monthly periods will return; the first bleed is therefore assumed to be abnormal. If you're on HRT, be wary of breakthrough bleeding at inappropriate times in the cycle. This is a symptom which still needs investigation.

Some common and non-serious causes of PMB are:

- polyps of the cervix or endometrium;
- trauma of intercourse after prolonged abstinence;

- atrophic vaginitis – due to lack of oestrogen 'drying up' vaginal tissues;
- fibroids – benign tumours of uterine muscle.

The serious causes of PMB are:

- cystic hyperplasia – over-growth of the endometrium due to excess stimulation with oestrogen. This can progress to endometrial cancer if not corrected;
- cervical cancer. This is usually picked up at an early stage by regular cervical smears, but PMB may be the first sign;
- endometrial cancer;
- ovarian cancer. Rarely, a hormone-secreting tumour may stimulate the womb and cause PMB.

If you experience any sort of vaginal bleeding that worries you, always consult your doctor. In the majority of cases, your mind will be put at rest. If there is a serious cause such as endometrial cancer, early treatment often results in a cure.

73. *When is it safe to stop using contraception after the menopause?*

Women nearing the menopause who wish to avoid pregnancy should use contraception for at least one year after their last period – so long as this takes them over the age of 50. If they are still under 50, contraception for a total of two years is advisable. If in doubt, your doctor can arrange a blood test to assess levels of FSH (follicle stimulating hormone). This will indicate whether contraception may cease.

MENOPAUSE

Fertility in a woman of 40 is half that of a woman in her 20s, and this falls even lower after the age of 45. The continuance of regular periods during the menopause indicates that around 95% will result in production of an egg. Irregular periods and episodes of 'missed' periods are more likely to indicate that ovulation is not occurring.

Most evidence suggests that modern, low-dose contraceptive pills may safely be used up to the age of 45 years in healthy, non-smoking women undergoing regular check-ups.

Smokers over 35 years face an increased risk of heart attacks and strokes if they remain on the pill. They are therefore advised to switch from the combined pill to the progestogen-only mini-pill, or to use other methods of contraception. Evidence linking the pill and breast cancer remains inconclusive and controversial.

The pill masks menopausal symptoms and it may not be clear, when a (non-smoking) woman stops it in her late 40s, whether or not she is fertile or post-menopausal. A blood test to measure Follicle Stimulating Hormone (FSH) a few months after stopping the pill will establish conclusively whether or not the menopause has arrived.

NB. HRT does *not* provide contraceptive protection.

The majority of pregnancies occurring over the age of 40 are unplanned. Obstetrical statistics show that the UK legal abortion rate for women over 40 years is 45% of the conception rate – that is, almost half the pregnancies are terminated.

The maternal mortality rate in the age group 40–49 is four times higher than for pregnant women aged 20–29, and the risk of death of the baby immediately before or after the birth is doubled as maternal age doubles. Chromosomal abnormalities in the foetus (for example Down's syndrome) are increasingly likely when a woman is over 35 years. The trauma of a therapeutic abortion may then have to be faced. Effective contraception is vital.

74. *What alternatives to HRT are available for treating menopausal symptoms?*

HRT is not the only option at the menopause. A healthy diet which is low in fat, high in calcium and vitamins, and followed in conjunction with regular exercise will decrease the risk of heart disease and osteoporosis.

Interestingly, according to a recent study, a diet high in fibre may result in a four-fold increase in mineral bone loss and accelerated osteoporosis. This may be due to minerals binding with fibre in the gut so that more is eventually excreted. This data is being evaluated further.

Menopausal flushing and headaches are helped by drugs that prevent dilation of blood vessels (clonidine, beta blockers). The avoidance of alcohol and caffeine is also beneficial.

Vaginal dryness, sexual discomfort and urinary symptoms may be treated with oestrogen creams applied locally to the skin, and results are often dramatic.

Relaxation techniques, homeopathy, acupuncture and other complementary disciplines have non-hormonal treatments to offer, and many women prefer these. However, they will not provide the same long-term benefits against heart disease.

75. *Why do women get osteoporosis?*

Bone consists of a network of collagen fibres filled with calcium salts. In osteoporosis, both components are lost, resulting in decreased bone density.

In the UK, 50,000 osteoporotic hip fractures occur every year. Fifty per cent of these patients are unable to continue living independent lives and every year, 6000 will die prematurely as a result of fracture complications.

Bone is a living tissue, constantly remodelling itself and responding to physical stress. This occurs through the coupled action of two sorts of cell: *osteoblasts*, which build bone, and *osteoclasts*, which absorb it. Peak bone mass is reached during ages 35–45 years, then bone density diminishes due to an imbalance between formation and resorption.

Bone is lost more rapidly in the ten years after the menopause, because of the loss of beneficial oestrogen effects on osteoblasts and osteoclasts.

The average post-menopausal woman loses 2–3% of her bone mass each year, but some lose up to 5%.

By the age of 70, untreated women will lose up to 30% of their pre-menopausal bone mass, and a few lose a staggering 50%. Those most at risk are women experiencing an early menopause before age 45, especially if this was due to hysterectomy and surgical removal of the ovaries.

Diet plays an important role in bone health. Low intakes of calcium *before* the menopause and low levels of vitamin A and D (which help absorption of calcium) have been shown to hasten osteoporosis. Cigarette smoking and heavy consumption of alcohol, coffee, meat and salt tend to reduce available calcium and are therefore associated with low bone density. Both anorexia nervosa and 'crash' dieting will increase loss of body calcium in the urine.

Immobility reduces mechanical stresses on bones and they respond by rapidly becoming porotic. Drugs such as steroids and some diseases (for example over-active parathyroid glands) also contribute to osteoporosis.

76. *Can osteoporosis be prevented?*

Prevention of future osteoporosis starts in childhood. Adequate intakes of calcium before puberty ensure maximal peak bone mass is achieved. Ninety-nine per cent of body calcium is stored in the bones. During pregnancy, lack of dietary calcium will result in minerals being leached from the mother's bones to build those of the foetus. Drinking plenty of milk (the richest source of calcium) is therefore important during pregnancy and while breast-feeding.

The greatest benefit in reducing osteoporosis and bone fractures are obtained by starting HRT at the menopause and continuing it for at least five years.

Increased weight-bearing physical activity and an adequate dietary calcium intake have beneficial effects, as do stopping smoking and keeping alcohol intake to moderate levels. A recent study in Cambridge suggests that small increases in vitamin D intake could increase average bone density levels and cut the number of fractures in women over 45.

MENOPAUSE

Vitamin D is made in small amounts by skin exposed to sunlight and is found in fish oils, dairy foods, eggs, liver and margarine. Interestingly, fluoride binds to bone and inhibits dissolution in the same way that it binds to teeth and hardens them against decay!

Cyclical treatment with etidronate disodium is now available as a non-HRT treatment for osteoporosis. It works by inhibiting osteoclasts, the cells responsible for bone resorption. The treatment is given in 90-day cycles with calcium supplementation so that normal bone formation and remodelling can continue unaffected. Over time, a net increase in bone mass and a marked reduction in the incidence of new vertebral fractures occur.

A hormone derived from salmon which can be delivered by injection (calcitonin) may be suitable for women unwilling or unable to take HRT. It regulates bone turnover and can increase bone density in post-menopausal women.

RECOMMENDED CALCIUM INTAKES
Boys: 1000 mg per day
Girls and pre-menopausal women: 800 mg per day
 (from age 11 years)
Pregnancy/breast-feeding: 1200 mg per day
Post-menopausal women: 1000 mg per day
Osteoporosis sufferers: 1000 mg per day

---

77. *Who should have bone density screening?*

Measurement of bone mineral density can accurately assess bone density in sites that matter most – the femoral head (hip) and lumbar vertebrae (spine).

WHAT WORRIES WOMEN MOST

However, there is controversy over the value of universal bone density screening.

One study estimated that bone screening would only prevent 5% of fractures in women, because less than a quarter of those invited would both attend for screening and then comply with any therapy (for example HRT, and the calcium-replacing drug, etidronate) prescribed.

Another study found that one in three menopausal women were at high risk of osteoporosis, which would make widespread screening desirable so long as treatment compliance could be improved. By the end of the first year, only 53% of those 'at risk' who had been prescribed HRT were still taking it – mainly because of returning periods. Prescription of tibolone, an HRT which doesn't usually cause menstrual bleeding, may improve these results.

Bone density screening cannot accurately distinguish between women who will go on to have a fracture in later life if not treated and those who will not. Two-thirds of fractures occur in women with bone densities above the lowest 20%, which limits screening effectiveness.

Fractures result from falls. Maintaining fitness, balance, alertness and eyesight in the elderly, providing walking aids, minimising medications likely to cause confusion or unsteadiness, and assessing safety in the home are all essential as preventive measures.

Reducing risk factors for osteoporosis in the general population by discouraging smoking, encouraging exercise and ensuring adequate dietary calcium – especially in children and pregnant/breastfeeding mums – may eventually prove more effective than widespread bone density screening.

Menopause

Current practice is to restrict screening to those known to be at risk of osteoporosis and not on HRT, for example: those with early menopause – especially if surgically induced; those on long-term steroid therapy; anorectics; and those with thyroid or parathyroid disease.

BREAST CANCER

Breast cancer and the thought of a mastectomy strike terror in any woman's heart. Breasts are vitally important to a woman's sense of self-image and femininity. Breast cancer strikes one woman in 11 and has been shown to have a hereditary component; whether this is due to environmental factors (for example a virus) or to genetic causes is unclear.

In any one year, 15,000 British women will die from this dreadful disease. In an attempt to fight back, they are encouraged to be 'aware' of their breasts and to detect subtle changes sooner rather than later. Early diagnosis and treatment of breast cancer has been shown to improve prognosis.

Modern therapy of breast cancer is less likely to be radical (surgical removal – mastectomy) and more likely to involve 'lumpectomy' with complementary treatments of radiotherapy, chemotherapy or the anti-oestrogen drug tamoxifen. This has greatly improved the psychological burden of serious breast disease.

78. *How should I check my breasts for lumps?*

British guidelines concerning self-examination of the breasts are currently in a state of chaos. Some specialists advise 'breast awareness' rather than formal self-examination, while others encourage regular breast examination according to a set protocol.

As long as you don't get obsessive and overly

BREAST CANCER

anxious, self-examination is at least something positive to do in the fight against serious breast disease. It only takes five minutes and, as 90% of breast tumours are discovered by women themselves, the more it is done routinely, the earlier cancers will be detected.

The important thing is to become familiar with the feel of your own breasts. Some are naturally more lumpy than others, but subtle changes can be detected.

Be aware of your breasts and examine them while bathing, showering and dressing. It is worthwhile for any woman over the age of 30 to set aside five minutes after each period (or once a month if she no longer gets them) to routinely check her breasts.

The following is a reasonable protocol.

Look at your breasts in a mirror and go through the following checklist with your arms by your sides, with arms raised above your head, and then with your hands firmly on your hips. With practice, it really doesn't take long:

- check that the outline of your breasts looks normal, with no change in size, shape or colour;
- examine your nipples. Are they the same shape? At the same level? Turning inwards? Scaling or reddening? Is there any discharge?;
- is there any puckering, dimpling or a rash?;
- are there any visible lumps or thickening?

Then lie down. Raise you left arm and rest it on a pillow behind your head. With your right hand, examine your left breast. Use the flat of the first three fingers (not the tips) and examine the breast using small, circular movements and firm pressure. Then bring the raised arm down by your side and continue feeling the same breast up as far as the collarbone and out into the armpit.

When you're happy that all is normal, raise your right arm and examine your right breast in the same way.

79. What should I do if I find a breast lump?

First, don't panic. Nine out of ten lumps are non-malignant, but all need investigation. In women under 30, most breast lumps are benign fibroadenomas ('breast mice'), but it is not easy to differentiate clinically between malignant and benign lumps. The classic description of cancer feeling 'hard and craggy' only applies in advanced cases. Microscopic examination of cells from all lumps is the safest option. Needle aspiration (inserting a fine needle and sucking up a few cells with a syringe) is the investigation of choice rather than surgical 'lumpectomy' and all the anguish this entails.

One in 11 women will develop a breast tumour. With odds like that, any breast changes discovered during self-examination should be discussed with your doctor straight away. Your GP would much rather see you, even if nothing is wrong, than have you neglect something potentially serious.

Even if you have discovered a cancer, think positive. Early diagnosis and treatment often result in a cure. A ten-year trial has found that self-examination cuts breast cancer deaths by 20%, as more cancers are detected at a non-invasive stage.

BREAST CANCER

80. What is a mammogram and who should have one?

In 1987, a £55 million nationwide British mammography programme was launched after it was discovered that the country had the highest rate of breast cancer in the world. A mammogram involves compressing a breast between two plates and taking a soft tissue X-ray. A survey of 600 women revealed that this was no more painful than giving blood, and two-thirds of women found it less uncomfortable than expected. Despite this, a third of women eligible for mammography are not taking up the offer due to expectations of pain.

Screening mammography is available in Britain on the NHS for all women over 50 years – and for those under that age in whom a surgeon thinks it necessary (that is, when there is breast cancer in the family).

Mammography detects cancers on average two years earlier than 'discovery by chance' and can reduce breast cancer deaths by one-third. However, some specialists believe this X-ray procedure carries risks of its own. A Canadian study showed a higher death rate from breast cancer in women under the age of 50 who had undergone mammography. No plausible explanation has been offered as to why this procedure is harmful for women under 50 but benefits those over this age.

Other specialists believe this particular study was flawed, pointing out that eight in ten women whose breast cancer was treated at the earliest stage were still alive five years later, while undetected tumours are responsible for eight out of ten deaths. Yet another recent study has found that women under the age of 50 who had a mammography-detected tumour had a five-year survival rate of 95%, compared with 74% in women whose tumours were detected manually, presumably at a later stage.

The dosage of radiation received during a mammogram is very low. Current best advice is – if you are offered a mammogram, take up the invitation. It makes sense that if you detect cancers early, the chances of successful treatment are better.

81. What causes breast pain?

Breast pain (mastalgia) is surprisingly common. Sixty-six per cent of working women in Cardiff admitted experiencing symptoms but few consulted their GP. It is important to remember that pain is not a common symptom of breast cancer, though this should always be excluded. Mastalgia can be divided into two groups – cyclical and non-cyclical.

Cyclical pain is usually present in both breasts but is often worse on one side. It improves when menstruation starts but may be continuous, only lessening during a period. It is often associated with lumpiness of the breasts and is usually worse in the second half of the menstrual cycle. This combination of cyclical breast pain and lumpiness is often labelled 'chronic mastitis' but it is neither infective nor inflammatory. Antibiotics are not needed, but are often prescribed.

Causes include hormonal imbalance; enzyme deficiency; fluid retention and pre-menstrual syndrome;

BREAST CANCER

over-sensitivity of breast tissue to hormones; and adenosis – an increase in the number and size of lobules in the breast.

Reducing saturated fats in your diet will help. These are broken down in the body to form hormone precursors, or prostaglandins. These may be responsible for triggering cyclical breast pain. Oil of evening primrose supplies gamolenic acid. This corrects hormonal imbalance in the breast. Taken in a dose of 3 gm per day, oil of evening primrose produces a good response in 70% of sufferers. It needs to be taken for at least three months before deciding how effective it is.

Other treatments include drugs to correct hormonal imbalances (for example danazol, tamoxifen, bromocriptine, goserelin).

Non-cyclical breast pain is not related to menstruation. Many cases are caused by cramping of the muscles between the ribs. Other causes include breast abscess, discharging and inflamed breasts, arid duct dilatation.

Post-menopausal women may experience non-cyclical mastalgia after starting HRT, but this usually subsides spontaneously.

COSMETIC BREAST SURGERY

It is increasingly acceptable for women to admit to having cosmetic surgery – not for reasons of vanity but as part of a spectrum of body improvement and care.

It has been estimated that over 2 million women have silicone breast implants in the USA, with 1.3 million operations performed for cosmetic purposes.

In the UK, around 100,000 women have undergone what is known as breast augmentation mammoplasty, of which half were performed for breast reconstruction after mastectomy, or for correction of gross asymmetry.

If you are considering any cosmetic operation, it is important to consult a properly trained practitioner. Contact the British Association of Aesthetic Plastic Surgeons, Royal College of Surgeons, Lincoln's Inn Fields, London WC2A 3PN, sending a stamped addressed envelope to obtain a list of accredited specialists.

82. Can breasts easily be made larger or smaller?

From a technical point of view, breast augmentation or reduction is not difficult. The skill lies in knowing exactly how far to go – and in obtaining symmetrical results.

With augmentation, size selectors are placed inside bras to assist pre-operative selection of the

COSMETIC BREAST SURGERY

new breast volume required. Incisions are made in the armpits and a silicone implant is inserted beneath the breasts.

Small breasts often droop and may require 'mastopexy' – lifting and repositioning of the nipple – in addition to augmentation. A circular scar will run around the areola (pigmented area round the nipple) and vertically down to meet a horizontal scar in the skin crease below the breast. Nipples are repositioned and sexual sensation and ability to breast-feed are usually preserved.

Breast reduction also involves relocation of the nipple and produces similar scars to mastopexy. These progressively fade and are not visible when wearing low-cut dresses or bikinis.

After a breast implant or reduction operation, provided the radiologist is warned, it is still possible to have a mammogram performed.

83. Do breast implants cause cancer?

In January 1992, the US Food and Drug Administration imposed a 45-day moratorium, or emergency ban, on the insertion of all breast implants. When this expired on February 19th, they advised continued use of implants only in certain circumstances and under supervision. Effectively, they have restricted access to implants in America until further research into safety is available. This has resulted in falling sales and at least one US breast implant manufacturer withdrawing from the market.

Despite media hype, breast implants have not convincingly been associated with increased risk of breast cancer. In 1990, an independent UK committee reviewed all available evidence concerning possible connections between silicone breast implants and increased incidence of cancer. They concluded there was nothing to support a link.

In 1991, manufacture of implants coated with polyurethane foam ceased due to a theoretical risk of polyurethane breaking down in the body to 2,4-toluene diamine (TDA) – a substance known to cause cancer in rats. There is no direct evidence, however, for the release of TDA from implants into humans (or animals).

Research has shown that, far from increasing the risk of breast cancer, straightforward augmentation mammoplasty may actually reduce it. One study, involving over 3000 women, expected to find 36 cases of breast cancer over a period of ten years. In fact, only 24 occurred. A second study in Alberta, involving almost 12,000 women, confirmed this statistically significant finding. It is possible that this reduced risk is due to the smaller mass of breast tissue present in women requesting implants, but this remains unclear.

The important implication is: there is no convincing evidence of increased risk of breast cancer in women who have had breast implants inserted.

84. *Do breast implants cause auto-immune disease or other problems?*

Following insertion of silicone gel breast implants, silicone micro-particles have been detected in lymph nodes (glands) and tissues elsewhere in the body.

COSMETIC BREAST SURGERY

They trigger an immune reaction with local formation of foreign-body 'granulomas', which are inflammatory changes in the tissue. These are characterised by 'giant cells' containing many nuclei. At the moment, there is no convincing evidence that silicone particle shedding from implants and their subsequent movement to other parts of the body has harmful results.

Some specialists say the giant cell reaction is among the most benign of inflammatory reactions the human body can mount against foreign substances. Others are more concerned, and have suggested that silicone migration increases the likelihood of connective tissue and auto-immune diseases, for example SLE (systemic lupus erythematosis), polymyositis (inflammation of muscles), Raynaud's syndrome (when extremities are cold), rheumatoid arthritis and scleroderma (hardening of connective tissues).

Current best advice is: it is unwise for a woman with pre-existing auto-immune disease, or a strong family history of it, to have a breast implant inserted.

For those concerned about the safety of silicone gel, other implants are available. Some are filled with salt solutions and others with plastic foam.

Perhaps the most distressing side-effect of breast implants is 'capsular contraction'. The body naturally walls off any foreign implant with a layer of fibrous scar tissue. This can contract and become so hard that eventually, when a woman lies down, her breasts do not fall to the side. Various studies have reported an incidence of capsular contraction from 3% to 76%. The majority of women, however, seem

What Worries Women Most

delighted with results after augmentation surgery – even if the implants harden.

All operations carry risks. Problems possible with breast surgery include bleeding; infection; hardening of implants; breast discomfort; silicone leakage; thickening of scars; poor symmetry.

Contrary to popular belief, breast implants do not explode in low-pressurised aeroplanes; nor do they cause problems for deep-sea divers!

THE AGEING SKIN

Wrinkles are one of the most obvious external manifestations of age. The skin (epidermis) retains its ability to control water evaporation but supporting tissues beneath atrophy and sag. Collagen fibres become matted and elastin fibres thicken, twist and branch so skin loses its resilience and elasticity. Over the decades, there is a massive accumulation of degenerative material. Without elastic properties, skin sags and cannot snap back into place after stretching. Sun exposure causes small veins to become sparse, dilated and disorderly. Some fine blood vessels disappear altogether and lack of blood drainage gives skin its sallow, dull tone. Interestingly, it is estimated that 75% of the total lifetime dose of damaging ultra-violet radiation is accumulated before the age of 20 from a childhood of playing in the sun!

There are three main types of wrinkle:

- crinkles – very fine wrinkles that disappear when skin is stretched. They are associated with elastic fibre deterioration which starts at around the age of 30;
- glyphic wrinkles – accentuations of normal skin markings. Skin becomes diffusely thickened and yellowed, especially in areas exposed to light, for example the neck and around the eyes;

WHAT WORRIES WOMEN MOST

- linear furrows – grooves related to long-standing animation patterns (expressions) of facial muscles. Their positions are determined in childhood.

85. Why do I get wrinkles?

Wrinkles are a normal part of the biological ageing process which can be modified by hereditary, hormonal and environmental factors.

The commonest cause of wrinkles is exposure to sunlight (photo-ageing). Up to 90% of age-associated cosmetic problems are due to ultra-violet damage, yet still we strive for that sexy, golden tan!

Certain light wavelengths (for example UVA and UVB) interfere with normal cell division. Cells cannot regenerate and immune defence mechanisms malfunction. Skin that is exposed to sun for long periods of time becomes thickened, yellowed, scaled and deeply wrinkled, with a high risk of developing skin cancer.

Premature wrinkling is associated with smoking. Heavy smokers are five times more likely to have facial wrinkles than non-smokers – and the number of wrinkles increases in direct relation to the number of cigarettes smoked.

86. What are collagen injections?

Collagen is the structural protein from which gelatin is derived. It is similar in many species, and the collagen used for human implantation is extracted and purified from cow skin. The first injections were performed in 1976 and since then, almost one

THE AGEING SKIN

million people have been treated in more than 20 countries.

Collagen is injected through a very fine needle together with a local anaesthetic. The solution plumps out wrinkles but is naturally re-absorbed over a period of three to 18 months; the injections need to be repeated fairly regularly. There is a risk of developing allergic reactions. Collagen injections are used to camouflage creases, furrows and scars – including the pockmarks of quiescent acne. Implants are also used to augment natural contours and create looks such as the pouting 'Paris Lip'.

Latest techniques involve vacuum-extraction of fat from your own buttocks (liposuction) which is then 'grafted' by injection into wrinkles. Re-absorption is slower than with collagen, so cosmetic results last longer. In the USA, 300,000 women a year have fat harvested in this way. The first 'fat bank' is to be established for young women to store 50 cubic centimetres of 'buttock extract' against the future development of cellulite and wrinkles!

Injection of textured silicone (bioplastique) into wrinkles is now also available. Unlike collagen injections, this is permanent but can only be used on certain sorts of lines. The skills needed for both liposuction and bioplastique are those of a fully trained reconstructive surgeon, otherwise results can prove disastrous.

WHAT WORRIES WOMEN MOST

87. Does the anti-wrinkle treatment tretinoin really work?

Tretinoic acid (tretinoin) has undergone controlled testing and has been shown to significantly reverse the effects of skin ageing. A 16-week trial showed overall improvement in wrinkling, pinkness and skin texture where tretinoin was applied to face and forearms but no improvement in control areas treated with plain cream. It took 2–4 months for improvement in fine wrinkling to show. American patients have used tretinoin for over two years and showed improvement in both fine and coarse wrinkling and sagging of skin around the eyes. In the UK, tretinoin is only licensed for clinical use in acne but it is available in some cosmetic preparations.

Tretinoin is a derivative of vitamin A. It probably works by binding to specific receptors which then interact with DNA (the nuclear genetic material) and affect the working of certain genes.

Skin and fibre cells become more active in their secretion of support substances into intercellular spaces. These include molecules which can bind up to 1000 times their own weight in water. This results in plumping up of skin wrinkles. Blackheads and pustules are also lifted upwards and outwards, hence the beneficial effect in acne. Tretinoin stimulates fibre cells to synthesise more collagen and superficial veins to dilate and proliferate. This improves oxygenation, and skin thickness can increase by up to 80%.

THE AGEING SKIN

American dermatologists feel tretinoin isn't working properly unless patients experience periodical skin peeling and occasional burning, redness and itching similar to sunburn. This is due to high local concentrations of vitamin A.

There are some theoretical worries about tretinoin causing cancer, but in fact it is used clinically as a treatment for both pre-malignant skin conditions and some skin tumours (for example basal cell cancer, and dysplastic naevi – the abnormal moles). Tretinoin has been available for 20 years and used in millions of acne patients. There have been no reports of increased production of skin tumours. Nevertheless, patients receiving tretinoin therapy are advised to use sunblocks and to avoid exposure to sunbeds.

88. What happens during a face-lift?

Face-lifts have been described as the only guaranteed way to turn back the biological clock, though they don't stop it ticking! Over 10,000 people per year in the UK have a face-lift, of whom 5% are men (30% male in America).

Surgical technique and skill are obviously important in determining how long the face-lift will last, but a good one should give ten years' satisfactory wear. Many surgeons recommend resculpturing eyes at the same time, as bags are more ageing than sagging skin elsewhere.

Face-lifts vary in their complexity. Mini 'lunch-hour' lifts involve tightening the skin with tucks behind the ears. The Sub-cutaneous Musculo-Aponeurotic System (SMAS) lifts deeper muscle as well as skin and gives a more natural, less tense look.

Recent advances are the Sub-Periosteal 'mask' Face-lift in which all soft facial tissues are stripped from the bone before lifting, and the Deep Plane Face-lift where muscles are actually repositioned. This avoids tightness by putting skin and muscles back where they were ten years previously.

Eye operations are done under general or local anaesthetic and involve cutting out excess skin and fat. Incisions are placed in skin creases and when healed should be virtually undetectable. Post-operatively, stitches are removed at three to five days and bruising and swelling usually resolve within two weeks.

The way patients treat their new, taut face is vital. Scars should be massaged with vitamin E cream and skin should be completely shielded from sunlight for six months; it will be unusually sensitive through having been stretched so thin.

Remember that all operations can go wrong. Scars can become thickened and infection can set in, and in severe cases, soft tissues and muscles may be lost. Nerves can be damaged or cut, leading to facial drooping. Make sure your surgeon is a fully trained cosmetic specialist by contacting the British Association of Aesthetic Plastic Surgeons at the Royal College of Surgeons, London.

89. What causes stretch marks?

Stretch marks are crease-like breaks in the skin known as striae. They are caused by ruptures in the subdermal layers where thinning and stretching has occurred. Gaining and losing weight rapidly (for example due to pregnancy) is a common cause.

The Ageing Skin

Young girls may notice stretch marks around their breasts at puberty if a rapid increase in cup size occurs. Some women escape them, however, even after multiple pregnancies, though no-one really knows why.

Striae are usually skin-coloured, but if they are due to excessive hormones (for example steroid drug side-effects; Cushing's disease – when the body secretes too much steroid; progesterone in pregnancy) they may be a reddish-purple. With time, they fade to a silvery grey.

Stretch marks are notoriously difficult to treat, as they often cover a wide area. Collagen injections or re-implantation of fat sucked from the buttocks will help disguise small areas.

Massage, homeopathy and aromatherapy have more to offer in prevention of stretch marks than traditional medicine. Essential oils to try include Rose Bulgar, Lavender and Tangerine mixed in a base of almond and wheatgerm oil.

Oil massage should be done at least once a day (for example during pregnancy) and should involve all areas where stretching occurs – thighs, buttocks, breasts and abdomen. Regular exercise to tone muscles will also prevent drooping, which always emphasises striae.

90. What can be done about excess body hair?

Hairiness is more common than people think. One-quarter of all women have noticeable hair on their face, 15% have hair on their chest, 30% have it on their lower abdomen and 40% on their thighs. Surprised? That's because the majority of British women practise either depilation or bleaching. The hairy female armpit is a rare sight indeed.

Facial hair increases after the menopause. By the age of 65, 40% of women have a noticeable moustache and 10% sprout hair on their chins. This is not due to any medically significant hormonal imbalance, but to a natural fall in oestrogen levels. Testosterone therefore exerts its action more effectively.

Cosmetic removal of hair (shaving, removal creams, plucking, epilation, waxing, sugaring abrasion) is only temporary. Contrary to popular belief, shaving does not thicken hair or even make it grow faster. It merely slices off the tapered tip of the hair shaft so that it feels flattened and stubbly.

Electrolysis can be permanent but only works on growing hair, not on follicles in their resting phase. Shaving a few days before treatment allows only growing hairs to be zapped, as resting ones will remain flush with the skin. A good electrologist is needed, as electrolysis from a less skilled practitioner can scar.

Waxing can be uncomfortable and may result in a pimply look reminiscent of a plucked goose. This can be helped by taking an aspirin or ibuprofen anti-inflammatory tablet half an hour before treatment. Two other methods are available: one is bleaching the hair, and the other is 'sugaring' the leg and then pulling the hair off like waxing.

Several drugs are available to minimise hairiness. They help 70% of sufferers, but take up to a year to achieve their full effect. An oral contraceptive pill is

THE AGEING SKIN

perhaps the most effective. One brand is especially formulated for women with excess hair or acne – both of which are testosterone effects.

ACNE

91. Why do I get spots?

Acne is a universal problem. Seventy per cent of teenagers get spots of some kind, and some will continue to suffer into their 30s and 40s.

A spot is an inflamed blackhead. During adolescence, sebaceous glands in the skin are activated under the influence of hormones and excessive oil (sebum) is secreted. Skin cells rapidly divide and often produce so many daughter cells that the opening of a hair follicle gets blocked. This traps freshly produced sebum inside and results in formation of a classic, enlarging blackhead (comedone). Contrary to popular belief, its dark colour is due to accumulation of the tanning pigment, melanin, and not to a build-up of dirt.

Changes in the acid level of the skin encourage growth of bacteria, and infection results in spots. Hereditary factors seem to play a part. There is little scientific evidence that fatty foods, dairy products or chocolate contribute to acne, but a low fat diet full of fresh fruit and vegetables does appear subjectively to improve skin clarity.

Certain cheap, greasy cosmetic creams are 'comedogenic' and encourage the formation of blackheads. It is worth investing in a dermatologically tested brand if your skin is prone to problems.

Hormonal changes do affect the skin. Some blends of contraceptive pill encourage spots and women often find their skin is most inflamed before a period.

ACNE

Try not to pick or squeeze your spots, as this forces bacteria further into the skin and aggravates the problem. It can even result in spreading infection, pits and scars.

92. What treatments are available for acne?

It is important to treat acne early, before scarring and pitting results. Unfortunately, in severe cases, six months' treatment may be needed before obvious improvement occurs. Compliance and perseverance are essential.

Mild cases often improve dramatically with dab-on antibiotic solutions. Moderate acne, where face and back are involved, usually requires oral antibiotics plus or minus local solutions for the face.

Women who also require contraception can be prescribed a special blend of the pill containing cyproterone acetate. This counteracts excess testosterone levels which are thought to be partly at fault.

In severe cases of acne, where scarring has already occurred, referral for specialist treatment can usually be arranged. Peeling agents, skin abrasives, laser therapy and even collagen injections may be used to even out pits. Cysts respond well to treatment with oral retinoids (vitamin A derivatives – prescribed by a specialist only under close supervision). Alternatively, cysts can be surgically removed or injected with steroids.

Topical retinoid treatment is licensed for acne use in this country (see Question 87). Retinoic acid (tretinoin) acts by stimulating division of fibre-making cells deep in the skin. This proliferation helps push spots up and out, to such an extent that

WHAT WORRIES WOMEN MOST

initially the skin may appear worse – lumpy and inflamed – before improving dramatically. Excessive use results in thin, shiny, red skin with soreness and peeling.

HEALTHY DIET

There is currently a tremendous amount of interest in the food on our plates. The old saying 'we are what we eat' is increasingly proving to be true.

In 1990 the Office of Population Censuses and Surveys took a major look at British eating habits. We obtain an average 42% of daily energy from dietary fat – with 16% of calories eaten in saturated form. This is far too high and partly accounts for the UK's position near the top of the coronary heart disease (CHD) league table.

Coronary heart disease is the commonest cause of death in Britain, with 180,000 victims succumbing every year. The process involved is atherosclerosis (clogging up of the arteries) and is directly related to the amount and types of fat (lipids) in our diet.

Women are in a better position than men. Oestrogen protects women against CHD by altering the types of fat in our blood, and possibly by a direct action on coronary artery walls. After the menopause, our risk of heart disease rapidly equals that of men – unless HRT is prescribed; oestrogen supplements then maintain our level of protection.

CHD is 90% less prevalent in Japan and most of Europe, where diets contain less fat of the saturated kind. In the under-developed Third World, coronary heart disease is virtually unknown.

93. What is cholesterol and what is a safe blood level?

Cholesterol is a type of fat unique to the animal kingdom. It forms the major component of cell membranes and is essential for the proper functioning of nerves, a healthy, water-resistant skin and the rapid healing of wounds. Cholesterol is also a vital building block in the manufacture of bile acids and steroid hormones (for example oestrogen, progesterone, testosterone).

Cholesterol travels around the body in the blood, where it is made soluble by joining up with protein carriers (lipoproteins). It exists in several forms, of which low- and high-density lipoproteins (LDL and HDL) are the most important. LDL is linked with heart disease as it is small enough to pass into artery walls and accumulate in atherosclerotic plaques.

It is estimated that lowering our average blood cholesterol level by only 10% will prevent a quarter of the 180,000 CHD deaths occurring in Britain each year.

It is important not to confuse 'pre-formed' cholesterol in the diet with HDL and LDL cholesterol in the blood. Most blood cholesterol is manufactured in the liver from dietary saturated fat. Eating pre-formed cholesterol (for example meat, eggs, oysters and other shellfish) has little overall effect on blood cholesterol levels. To lower our LDL cholesterol we must cut down on dietary saturated fat.

Ideally, all adults should have their blood cholesterol level measured once before the age of 30. It is

HEALTHY DIET

especially important for males, or for those of either sex who smoke, are overweight, have high blood pressure, diabetes or a personal or family history of chest pains, heart attack or hyperlipidaemia (high fat levels in the blood). Estimation is best done while fasting, that is, first thing in the morning before anything is eaten or drunk.

Most blood tests measure total cholesterol levels. If these prove high, it is important to estimate the ratio of HDL and LDL in the blood. If most cholesterol is in the form of LDL, the risk of coronary heart disease is high. If most cholesterol is in the form of HDL, risk of hardening of the arteries (atherosclerosis) and CHD is less.

BLOOD CHOLESTEROL LEVEL CLASSIFICATION (British Hyperlipidaemia Association):

Desirable	less than 5.2 mmol/l
Borderline	5.2–6.4 mmol/l
Abnormal	6.5–7.8 mmol/l
High	more than 7.8 mmol/l

'NORMAL' LIMITS FOR VARIOUS BLOOD LIPIDS (various sources):

Total cholesterol	less than 5.2 mmol/l
Triglycerides	less than 2.3 mmol/l
LDL cholesterol	less than 3.5 mmol/l
HDL cholesterol	more than 1 mmol/l

Less strict criteria apply for pre-menopausal women.

Stricter criteria apply to men under 30 and all patients with CHD.

WHAT WORRIES WOMEN MOST

If your blood cholesterol level is above 6.4 mmol/l you will be advised to follow a low-fat, cholesterol-lowering diet. If your blood level is dangerously high, you may be prescribed lipid-lowering drugs.

Interestingly, it has been shown that eating 3 g or more of soluble fibre from oats (roughly equal to two large bowls of porridge) per day can lower total blood cholesterol levels by up to 0.16 mmol/l. This is a small, but significant change.

94. How much fat should my diet contain?

The Committee on Medical Aspects of Food Policy (COMA) recommend that we lower the fats in our diet to 35% of calories, with no more than 11% being saturated. American guidelines go even further. They recommend eating no more than 30% of total food energy as fat, with 10% or less being saturated. (This can easily be worked out using ready-reckoners available in most newsagents.) Don't, however, reduce your total fat intake to below 20% of calories, despite the current trend towards very low fat diets. You might run into problems with fat deficiency.

The fat in our diet comes in several forms including saturated, mono-unsaturated, and poly-unsaturated. Saturated fat is the 'baddie'. This is converted in our liver to a form of cholesterol (Low Density Lipid – LDL) which is small enough to seep from the blood into artery walls. It accumulates in swellings known as 'plaques' and encourages the formation of blood clots (thrombosis). As these accumulations grow larger, they block arteries totally or break off and travel round the body in the

HEALTHY DIET

bloodstream. Both events are serious and can result in angina, heart attacks, strokes, clots on the lung and even death.

Saturated fats are also processed to form a particular series of prostaglandins (hormone-like chemicals, for example thromboxane) which increases the stickiness of blood and encourages constriction of blood vessels. This makes sluggish circulation and thrombosis more likely.

Easy ways to lower the amount of saturated fat in your diet include:

- replacing butter and cream with mono-unsaturated products derived from olive oil, or with poly-unsaturates;
- switching to low-fat brands of mayonnaise, salad dressing, cheese, milk, yoghurt, etc;
- eating less red meat. Three times per week or less is better than the more usual once or twice per day. Trim all visible fat from meat and try to buy lean cuts;
- having regular vegetarian days – but don't over-indulge in hard cheese or eggs;
- eating more fish;
- avoiding foods high in saturated fat such as coconut, creamy soups, chocolate, pâté, oysters, prawns;
- cutting down on cakes, chips, biscuits and crisps;
- grilling rather than frying;
- eating baked potatoes rather than roasted or chipped.

Eighty-five per cent of the British population are eating more saturated fats than advised. Experiments show that by following a low-fat regime, plaque deposits on arterial walls start to diminish. It is never too late to adjust your diet and greatly improve your heart's health.

95. Is the Mediterranean diet really good for the heart?

Yes. The so-called Mediterranean diet (high in olive oil, fish, white meat, vegetables, fruit, bread, pasta, rice, alcohol and vitamins C and E but low in salt, sugar, red meat and saturated fat) has consistently been proven beneficial for the heart. Blood fat changes from adopting the Mediterranean diet take up to 14 days to appear, but reduced risk of heart disease lasts for years providing you stick to the diet.

Olive oil is beneficial to the heart as it is high in mono-unsaturated fat (oleic acid). This has a blood cholesterol-lowering effect.

Fish oils are high in poly-unsaturated fat and eicosapentanoic acid (EPA). EPA is especially good for the heart.

Dietary EPA is processed in the human body to make HDL cholesterol and a different series of prostaglandins than are made by saturated fat (for example prostacyclin). These lower the stickiness of blood and encourage dilation of small blood vessels. This makes thrombosis and atherosclerosis less likely.

Research has shown that the benefits of the Mediterranean diet may also come from vitamins C and E which are found in olive oil, fruit and vegetables. These vitamins inhibit oxidation of LDL cholesterol and the uptake of breakdown

HEALTHY DIET

products by scavenger cells (macrophages). This makes atherosclerosis less likely. These protective effects may explain anomalies such as France having the lowest incidence of coronary heart disease in Europe, despite its reputation for excessive rich food, wine, strong cigarettes . . . and women!

Consumption of a moderate amount of alcohol (for example a couple of glasses of wine per day) has now been shown to have a protective effect against heart disease. The recommended safe weekly limit for women, however, is 14 units (140 g alcohol) and for men, 21 units (210 g alcohol).

SLIMMING

Current dieting methods are failing. The Great British public spend an annual £1000 million on slimming foods, books and magazines but despite this, 45% of men and 36% of women are overweight. Twelve per cent of women and 8% of men are clinically obese, with a Body Mass Index (BMI – see Question 96) of 30 or over.

Despite a decade of improved nutritional advice, and an average calorie intake *below* the recommended level, over the last ten years the incidence of being overweight has increased in the UK by 15% for men and 12% for women. Something somewhere is going drastically wrong. Healthy eating policies are simply not hitting home. Those under 35 years are eating more 'junk' foods such as pies, chips and burgers, and a significant number of men are obtaining a staggering 28% of their total energy intake in the form of alcohol.

After smoking, obesity is the main risk factor that can be tackled to lower the UK's coronary heart disease deaths.

96. *What is my 'ideal' weight?*

The traditional height/weight/frame charts drawn up by insurance companies were calculated from population 'norms' and we have already seen that it is now almost normal to be overweight.

These tables were at best haphazard and at worst, easily susceptible to cheating!

Quetelet's Body Mass Index is the recommended

SLIMMING

modern method to assess how overweight you are. It is obtained by dividing your weight (in kilograms) by the square of your height (in metres):

$$\text{BMI} = \frac{\text{Weight (kg)}}{\text{Height} \times \text{Height (m}^2)}$$

The calculation will produce a number that can be interpreted by the following table:

			PREVALENCE	
BMI	**WEIGHT BAND**	**GRADE**	**WOMEN**	**MEN**
less than 20	Underweight			
20–25	Healthy	0		
25–30	Overweight	I	24%	37%
30–40	Obese	II	12%	8%
more than 40	Morbidly obese	III	0.3%	0.1%

The occasional gremlin can affect results; for example, bodybuilders with excessive muscle mass may have a BMI of up to 30 without actually being obese.

A BMI of 20–25 is desirable as this is not associated with increased risk of death. If your BMI is approaching or exceeding 30 kg/m^2 you should seriously consider losing weight. Your chance of death doubles as BMI rises from 30 to 40 kg/m^2.

Many diseases which kill are closely related to excess fat, for example heart attacks, strokes, high blood pressure, diabetes and even cancer.

97. *How many calories do I need?*

The answer depends on your age, your sex and your general level of activity. Obviously a labourer will need more calories to maintain his weight than a clerk sitting quietly at a desk.

WHAT WORRIES WOMEN MOST

The old 'Recommended Daily Amounts' for calories were recently superseded by 'Dietary Reference Values' by the Committee on Medical Aspects of Food Policy (COMA 1991). They suggest the following intakes:

RECOMMENDED KILOCALORIES PER DAY (K Cals)

AGE	MEN	WOMEN
19–49	2550	1940
50–59	2550	1940
60–64	2380	1900
65–74	2330	1900
Over 75	2100	1810

These are only guidelines based on average activities. Have a look at the following chart to get some indication of the calories you burn every day by gardening, cycling, swimming, etc. If you are trying to lose weight, you need to eat 500–1000 calories below your normal daily calorie needs.

ACTIVITY	APPROXIMATE NUMBER OF CALORIES BURNED PER HOUR
Sitting	90
Standing	100
Driving a car	140
Walk (stroll)	180
Bowling	250
Gardening	250
Swimming	300
Golf	300

SLIMMING

Walk (brisk)	350
Dancing	350
Jogging	500
Tennis	500
Cycling	650

98. Why am I fat? Is it my hormones or my metabolism?

Excess weight results when energy intake exceeds energy output over a prolonged period of time. Being fat indicates that you have eaten more than you required over the years.

Hormones and metabolism sometimes play a part, as they help to determine how many calories you need. Some bodies are genetically 'wasteful' of calories and stay slim. Others transform food into glycogen and fat stores with exemplary efficiency. These are more prone to obesity, as studies with identical twins have shown.

From the age of 27, our metabolism starts to slow and we burn up fewer calories. Between the ages of 27 and 47, the metabolism may slow by as much as 12%. If exercise levels stay the same (and they usually decline as well!), calorie intake must also drop to avoid an increase in weight. A slowing metabolism which yields an excess 100 calories per day will result in an extra 5 kg of fat gained per year!

The thyroid gland helps to set our metabolic rate by secreting the hormone *thyroxine*. When too little is made, the metabolism slows and weight increases. This can be diagnosed by a simple blood test, and hormone supplements can be prescribed. If you are overweight and have had difficulty dieting in the past, it is worth asking your doctor to screen you for an underactive thyroid. If can be difficult to diagnose clinically and requires a blood test.

Other hormone problems causing obesity are rare. Your doctor would know very quickly if you were suffering from one of these.

99. What is the best way to lose weight?

The *only* way to lose weight is by eating fewer calories than you burn. It is best to achieve this slowly at a rate of 0.5–1 kg (1–2 lb) per week. If you lose weight more rapidly than this (crash dieting), fat tends to go back on very quickly. This is partly because the body learns to use energy economically. As soon as you revert to normal patterns of eating, every calorie will 'stick'.

If you have more than 6 kg (a stone) to lose, it is best to follow a regime of 1200–1500 calories per day. If you have less than 6 kg to lose, an intake of 1,000 calories per day will do the trick. Always weigh food – never rely on guessing when you're following a calorie-restricted diet.

Drink plenty of fluids and maintain an adequate intake of fibre. Fresh fruits, vegetables and salads will ensure you don't develop a nutrient deficiency. Above all, try to cut back on fats. Fats yield 9.5 calories per gram. Protein and carbohydrate contain only 4 calories per gram. Carbohydrates tend to be 'watered down', which reduces their calorie count even further. Buy a calorie and fat guide from a

SLIMMING

newsagent to calculate your intakes accurately (see Question 94).

Some dieters find success by giving up red meat and eating plenty of fish. Having two or three vegetarian days per week will help to shed those pounds and as a bonus makes your diet healthier for your heart.

100. Are slimming pills safe?

A variety of 'slimming pills' are available. They work in different ways and some are safer than others. Those you buy over the counter are 'bulking agents'. They swell in the stomach when water is added and make you feel full quickly. They work well for some people, especially at the beginning of a diet when hunger pangs can be vicious. Prolonged use, however, may lead to tolerance ('immunity') and will not help the modification of behavioural and eating habits that you must make.

Slimming pills have in the past received a bad press due to a few doctors prescribing mixtures of amphetamine (a stimulant), diuretics (which cause increased urination), thyroxine tablets and even tapeworm eggs in an attempt to help patients lose weight – usually in exchange for 'fat' fees!

A new class of drugs, 'serotoninergic agents', is giving hope and help to slimmers desperately struggling to lose weight. These work by fooling the brain into thinking you have already had a carbohydrate snack.

When we eat carbohydrate, a brain chemical called serotonin is released. This causes a feeling of well-being and is one of the reasons we tend to eat when we're depressed. It makes us feel good.

A serotoninergic drug, for example dexfenfluramine, releases serotonin so that the brain stops craving carbohydrate. Hunger pangs stop and we feel satiated (full). The drug acts as a 'diet selector'. The brain starts fancying cottage cheese salads and rejects stodgy foods such as doughnuts and chocolate eclairs! In this way, serotoninergic agents also help to retrain eating habits.

Most other slimming pills fall into the class of 'central nervous system stimulants' and have similar effects to amphetamines. They are potentially addictive and their use is strictly controlled. They may also cause psychiatric disturbances as a side-effect.

New research indicates there are exciting times ahead for dieters. 'Thermogenic' drugs which boost the metabolism and 'lipolysis inhibitors' that stop dietary fats being broken down are currently at the research stage.

101. Are Very Low Calorie Diets (VLCDs) safe?

VLCDs should only be undertaken with close medical supervision – usually in hospital. Occasionally they have a role to play, but nutritional content needs very careful calculation. VLCDs may be combined with procedures such as jaw wiring in cases where health is severely at risk from obesity, for example if BMI is over 40 kg/m^2.

Unsupervised VLCDs can result in the breaking down of protein in the body (ketosis), dehydration, salt imbalance, mental confusion and even coma. Heart muscle becomes weak and a few deaths have been reported. Essentially they are equivalent to the total exclusion diets followed by victims of anorexia nervosa and those on hunger-strike. They should only ever be used under close, professional supervision.

102. What causes bulimia or anorexia nervosa?

Eating disorders are conditions where food intake has become extreme, with either too much (bulimia nervosa) or too little (anorexia nervosa) being consumed. Both conditions, but especially bulimia, are characterised by self-induced vomiting and abuse of laxatives, diuretics or purgatives. While the focus seems to be on food, these disorders are expressions of deep psychological and emotional problems. Their causes are not simple, but eating disorders share a number of features:

- an overwhelming fear of becoming fat;
- a compulsive drive towards thinness;
- low self-esteem and self-worth judged on body shape and size;
- bizarre eating habits such as extreme dieting or bingeing, self-induced vomiting, vigorous exercise, inappropriate use of diuretics and purgatives;
- using eating or refusal to eat as emotional weapons and as a means of coping with stress.

Nine out of ten cases affect females and the majority start during the teens or early twenties. Approximately 1 in 150 girls aged 15 to 18 suffer from anorexia and 1–2% of women between 18 and 25 years of age suffer from bulimia.

If you diet sensibly and lose weight at a rate of 1 kg

WHAT WORRIES WOMEN MOST

per week you are unlikely to develop a serious eating disorder. If you are worried by any aspects of your eating behaviour, it is best to consult a doctor for referral to a behavioural therapist, sooner rather than later. Your health is definitely at stake.

103. Should I take vitamin pills?

Most people think of vitamins as being good for you – but what they don't realise is that too many can be just as bad as not enough. Vitamins are organic substances essential to the workings of the body but are only required in very small amounts.

Excess water-soluble vitamins (C and the B complex) will be excreted via the kidneys and liver; literally money down the drain if you're taking expensive pills you don't need.

Fat-soluble vitamins (A, D, E and K) cannot leave the body easily as they do not dissolve in water. They build up and may lead to poisoning. Vitamin A is especially dangerous. Five hundred cases of intoxication, with several deaths, have been reported. Chronic overdose can result from only ten times the recommended intake – leading to swelling of the brain, headache, vomiting, liver damage and problems with skin and bones. Foetal abnormalities may result.

Use vitamins pills sensibly. If you follow a healthy diet with plenty of fresh fruits and vegetables plus lean meat and fish, you'll be getting all the vitamins you need. Vegetarians and pregnant women may need vitamin supplements in certain circumstances. If in doubt, consult your doctor.

SLIMMING

104. How much exercise do I need?

Exercise improves your suppleness, strength and stamina. It helps the heart work more efficiently, and by improving your circulation, reduces your risk of coronary heart disease. By increasing the number of calories you burn, exercise will assist the weight loss process. By firming your muscles, it will improve your silhouette. You should try to exercise for at least half an hour, three times a week as a minimum. Begin gently and increase gradually, day by day if possible. Always warm up first. Make sure you are suitably clad for your chosen sport. Footwear is very important if you are walking or running – and if out at night, wear light colours and better still, fluorescent strips.

Walking is a good way to begin if you are really unfit. If you suffer joint problems such as arthritis, swimming and cycling are excellent as they don't involve weight-bearing on the hips and knees.

105. What operations can help me lose weight?

If you are seriously obese with a Body Mass Index of greater than 40 kg/m^2, your risk of death is 2.5–3 times that of a person of normal weight. You need to lose weight as a matter of urgency. Some sympathetic surgeons may be prepared to discuss the following operations:

- jaw wiring. This immobilises the upper and lower jaws by applying braces to the teeth. Nutrition is obtained via a straw. Usually, vitamin-enriched liquid food supplements are

prescribed, though 'normal' food may be liquidised and diluted;
- fundoplasty. This is a major operation in which the stomach is stapled. The resulting pouch can only hold half the usual volume. Feelings of fullness occur soon after eating. Food must be taken 'little and often' or vomiting may occur;
- liposuction. During this technique of 'spot reduction', fatty tissue is broken down by enzymes and literally sucked off the body. It tends to be used for cosmetic reasons only;
- apronectomy. This operation involves cutting away the overhanging skin from the anterior abdominal wall. It is useful for those who have lost a lot of weight and have ended up with an unsightly bag of loose abdominal skin. A prominent scar will result.

ALCOHOL

When it comes to solvent abuse, alcohol is the chemical of choice for many women. It is the most widely available drug in Britain and 90% of adults indulge – even if only occasionally. Alcohol enriches the palate of connoisseurs, lubricates social conversation and is the reason for many a party. In moderation, alcohol can even prolong your life. It is over-indulgence that causes harm.

According to the organisation Alcohol Concern, one in six women drink over the healthy limit and 200,000 women drink more than 35 units of alcohol per week. If done regularly, this will seriously damage their health.

106. How much can I safely drink?

Non-pregnant women may safely drink a maximum of 14 units of alcohol per week. Over 35 units per week is dangerous. The healthy limit for men is 21 units, with greater than 50 units being dangerous.

1 unit (10 g alcohol) = 100 ml (one glass) of wine
 = 50 ml (one measure) of sherry
 = 25 ml (single tot) of spirit
 = 300 ml (½ pint) of beer.

Most drinkers tend to overestimate the strength of spirits and underestimate the strength of beer; for example, a man drinking two pints of beer has consumed *four* units. A woman drinking two glasses

WHAT WORRIES WOMEN MOST

of wine and a double vodka has also consumed *four* units.

In pregnancy, more than 12 units of alcohol per *week* is associated with foetal growth retardation; more than 9 units per *day* is associated with the more serious foetal alcohol syndrome. This is characterised by low birth-weight babies, a high risk of stillbirth, abnormalities of the offspring's face (deformed ears, receding chin and forehead, upturned nose), congenital heart disease and low intelligence.

If possible, avoid alcohol altogether for the three months before conception and the first three months of pregnancy. During the last six months of pregnancy, one glass of wine per day may be enjoyed.

107. What effects does alcohol have on the body?

In moderation, alcohol is beneficial. It counteracts the effects of stress by promoting relaxation. Moderate drinkers have lower blood pressure than non-drinkers and are at less risk of a stroke. Alcohol also protects against coronary heart disease and lowers blood cholesterol levels.

Alcohol is a weak general anaesthetic, depressing all parts of the brain in a predictable order. The sequence of events is:

- tranquillisation (removal of anxiety);
- excitation (verbosity, recklessness);
- slurring of speech (dysarthria);
- staggering (ataxia);
- sedation (deep sleep).

ALCOHOL

The next stages lead to coma and death.

Alcohol is metabolised in the liver by specific enzymes at a rate of about 8 g/hour. If more than the safe limit is consumed, liver poisoning results. Initially, liver cells fight back by producing more alcohol-degrading enzymes. Levels of these in the blood give a good indication of how much someone is drinking. When this countermeasure fails, liver cells undergo fatty change and eventually cirrhosis results.

Cirrhosis is a serious disease where the liver becomes lumpy, fibrous and shrinks. Changes are mostly irreversible and frequently fatal due to haemorrhage or liver failure.

Excessive alcohol weakens heart muscle. Men who drink more than three pints a day (six units) are at twice the risk of sudden cardiac death than those drinking moderately (two to four units). Binge drinkers, and those who drink heavily only at weekends and holidays, are also more at risk.

Alcohol is a weak diuretic (increasing urination) and will lead to progressive dehydration. Women who drink moderately at the start of their period may experience a sudden flow of retained fluid.

108. What are the signs of alcohol dependency?

In excess, alcohol has devastating effects on our mental health and social behaviour.

Alcoholics have difficulty concentrating, become forgetful, irritable and secretive. They may stay out drinking for long hours and often get violent when

What Worries Women Most

confronted. Some get into debt, are a major cause of accidents, and jeopardise the stability of their family unit with their behaviour.

Although simplistic, the following guidelines may help pinpoint someone with a problem who needs help:

- drinks early in the day;
- always has alcohol close to hand;
- smells of alcohol at work;
- commits drink-driving offences;
- becomes angry when drinking habits are raised;
- has to increase alcohol intake to gain the same effect previously achieved with smaller amounts;
- feels sick, shaky, sweaty and 'hung-over' in the mornings;
- has lots of time off sick.

For more information, contact Alcohol Concern at 275 Gray's Inn Road, London WC1X 8QF. Tel: 071-833 3471.

SMOKING

There are around 14 million cigarette smokers in the UK, of whom two-thirds want to give up. Unfortunately this is easier said than done. Nicotine is addictive and withdrawal symptoms of tension, aggression, depression, insomnia and craving can occur. Of teenagers who decide to 'experiment' with just a few cigarettes, 90% become trapped in a long-term addiction to nicotine. Eighty per cent of smokers who try to give up, relapse within one year, leaving only 35% of smokers who succeed in quitting before the age of 60.

Twenty-nine per cent of all women smoke. They seem to need more help than men to give up, as women are more likely to smoke with the deliberate intention of curbing their appetite and controlling their weight. They are reluctant to abandon this effect. Women also use cigarettes to cope with negative feelings and to keep their hands occupied when nervous in social situations. Men, on the other hand, use cigarettes to enhance positive feelings when they are having a good time.

The number of smokers is beginning to fall, but fewer women than men are giving up. The number of male smokers fell from 35% in 1986 to 31% in 1990 but the number of women smokers only dropped from 31% to 29% over the same period.

Three hundred new smokers in the UK are hooked every day.

What Worries Women Most

109. Why is smoking unhealthy?

It has been shown conclusively from a study involving half a million people that the risk of early death in smokers is nearly double that of non-smokers. The most frequent age of death for female smokers is 85, while non-smoking women live on average to 91. In males, average age at death is reduced from 87 to 81 in smokers. Smoking cuts six years off your life and in addition, have a look at the following:

- 4000 different chemicals are present in tobacco smoke of which many are carcinogenic (cancer-forming);
- up to a quarter of all cot deaths are thought to be associated with passive smoking;
- passive smoking is involved in 4000 miscarriages per year;
- passive smoking causes asthma, eczema and glue ear in young children;
- smokers have 2.4 times the risk of depressive illness;
- smoking impairs the rigidity of penile erections, with a clear dose-related effect;
- brain haemorrhage is six times more likely in young smokers than non-smokers;
- infertility is three times more likely in smokers;
- smoking-related diseases kill 40% of smokers before retirement;
- because of the likelihood of an early demise, life insurance companies charge smokers 50% more than non-smokers;
- smoking during pregnancy causes malfunction

SMOKING

of the placenta, still-birth, low birth-weight babies and babies of lower intelligence;
- there are 300 deaths per day in the UK from smoking – doctors can now write 'smoking' as the cause of death on certificates.

Smoking causes angina; impotence; heart attack; high blood pressure; dilated aortic artery; stroke; chronic obstructive airways disease; stomach ulcers; senile dementia; abortion; blindness; wrinkles; cancer of the mouth, throat, breast, lung, pancreas, kidney, cervix and bladder. Many effects are due to the spasm and constriction of arteries and veins which occurs within seconds of each nicotine dose.

Yet ask any smoker what damage smoking does to the body and most will say it only affects the lungs. Within 48 hours of giving up smoking, levels of clotting factors in the blood fall low enough to reduce the chance of a heart attack or a stroke. Within a year, your risk of other diseases will also have come down to near-normal levels. It is therefore never too late to stop smoking to save your life.

110. What is the easiest way to stop smoking?

Some smokers find the easiest way to stop is to make the decision and just give up. Others require extensive counselling and rely on nicotine replacement to see them through.

A simple 'quit' plan might involve the following:
1. Name the day to give up and get into the right frame of mind.

WHAT WORRIES WOMEN MOST

2. Find support – giving up nicotine is easier with a friend or partner.
3. Save the money previously spent on cigarettes in an 'Ash Cash' fund. Decide on a luxury to buy with it. This could even be a holiday abroad, as an amazing amount of money per month can accumulate.
4. Throw away all smoking paraphernalia – papers, matches, lighters, ashtrays, spare packets.
5. Find a hobby to take your mind off smoking, and generally become more active. Take up regular exercise and improve your overall fitness.
6. Identify situations where you would usually smoke and either avoid them or plan ahead on how you will overcome them.
7. Be careful with your diet. Avoid excess saturated fats. Count calories so you do not put on weight. Chew sugar-free gum or drink water and diet drinks instead. Brushing your teeth will help control a craving.
8. Enrol someone to encourage you – to praise you when you are doing well. Psychological tricks like this sound ridiculous – but they work. Keep a 'star chart' and stick a gold star in a booklet for every cigarette-free day. Plan a reward for every week of success.
9. Learn to relax. Join a health club and wallow in the sauna or whirlpool. Have a massage, practise yoga or meditation. You need something to replace the anxiety-reducing effects of nicotine.

If you find the going tough, consider using nicotine replacement products such as skin patches or

SMOKING

chewing-gum. Alternative medicine can also help. Hypnotherapy, acupuncture, aromatherapy and relaxation therapy have succeeded where will-power has often failed.

PSYCHIATRY

Anxiety and depression are closely linked and 15% of the population suffer one or the other each year. The lifetime risk of developing severe depression is between 8 and 12% for men, between 20 and 26% for women. Female incidence is higher because of the emotional effect of hormonal swings occurring after childbirth (post-natal depression) and around the menopause.

Recently, two new types of depression have been recognised. Seasonal Affective Disorder (SAD) and Recurrent Brief Depression (RBD).

RBD is believed to affect six million people in the UK. It is characterised by brief bouts of depression lasting two or three days, which suddenly lift. It can affect sufferers up to 20 times per year and tends to strike suddenly. It is thought to be due to changes in brain activity and as yet, there is no satisfactory drug treatment. It is possible that there is a link between this condition and pre-menstrual syndrome.

Seasonal affective disorder (SAD) is related to changing seasons. As days get shorter and nights draw in, its incidence increases. Very little is known about this form of depression but the light-sensitive pineal gland in the brain is thought to play a role.

111. What are the symptoms of stress?

Stress is a socially acceptable form of anxiety. The physical and mental symptoms are the same but the 'diagnosis' is less embarrassing.

PSYCHIATRY

Some stress is good for us – it makes us competitive, steers us through difficult situations and pushes us towards our goals. Too much, however, can be harmful.

Excess stress causes secretion of adrenaline in a primitive 'fight or flight' reaction. Blood flows to our muscles and away from our brain. Blood pressure is raised, arteries constricted, and coronary artery spasm, sudden heart attack or even a stroke can result.

The physical symptoms of stress are numerous and include tiredness; insomnia; sweating; flushing; palpitations; skipped heartbeats; rapid pulse; dizziness; faintness; pins and needles; numbness; headaches; abdominal pain; nausea; diarrhoea; frequency of passing urine; chest pain; and angina.

Mental indicators of stress can be more distressing and include overwhelming feelings of anxiety and panic; fear of rejection; fear of failure; loss of ability to concentrate; loss of libido; impotence; reliance on alcohol, smoking or drugs; obsessive and compulsive behaviour; feelings of isolation from colleagues and friends; a sense of impending doom. Suicide may even result.

Many of the above symptoms will be experienced by the average adult on a regular basis.

112. How can I lower my stress levels?

Stress comes from two main sources: from within an individual (unfitness, disruption of biorhythms, negative self-image, personality type) and from the environment (change, uncertainty over employment

WHAT WORRIES WOMEN MOST

or finance, changes in relationships, bereavement, unrealistic goals, etc).

Psychologists recommend the following game plan as the best way of adapting to stress:

- improve levels of fitness and eat a healthy diet. Avoid excess alcohol, nicotine, caffeine and drugs;
- channel aggression into activities such as non-competitive sport;
- learn relaxation techniques. Set aside frequent periods of time for relaxation ('quality time');
- work out which situations and people induce stress, and avoid them;
- identify your good points. Improve your bad ones, then accept them as part of you. Try not to be a perfectionist;
- don't compare yourself unfavourably with others;
- don't expect others to change before you are prepared to change yourself;
- set realistic goals and tackle big problems one step at a time;
- expect to make mistakes, apologise and learn from them;
- learn to be patient, for example let the pushy so-and-so with the Porsche into the traffic queue ahead of you; don't jump red lights. Instead of swearing in a traffic jam, keep a bottle of soapy water to hand and blow bubbles out of the window.
- talk more slowly and listen to others without interrupting;

PSYCHIATRY

- formulate decisions in unhurried circumstances and not under deadline pressure;
- be assertive. Say 'no' and mean it. An unreasonable request is not made more reasonable by your squandering time fulfilling it;
- inject a positive thought – a 'Meichenbaum' – into your day as an antidote to stressful situations: for example, 'Every day, in every way, I get better and better.' This certainly helped Inspector Dreyfus in *The Pink Panther*!

Vitamin C and the B complex are depleted during stress as they are used in the adrenaline-mediated 'fight or flight' response. Vitamin B is further depleted by metabolising alcohol and sugary foods resorted to under stress, so supplements may be warranted. Eat little and often to maintain blood sugar levels, eat high-fibre wholefoods, and decrease intake of sugar, salt and saturated fats. Above all, learn to relax. As well as improving your attitude to life, it may well succeed in prolonging it.

113. What can be done about anxiety?

Anxiety affects 5% of the population and is associated with feelings of apprehension, dread and impending doom. Short-lived anxiety is appropriate in some situations, for example weddings, examinations or flying, but those with morbid anxiety worry excessively about trivial matters. They experience severe symptoms of an over-active nervous system: restlessness, palpitations, tremor, flushing, dizziness, hyperventilation, loose bowels, sweating, muscle tension and insomnia, etc. Symptoms are identical to those induced by stress, for stress is an anxiety state. Depression often accompanies anxiety as well.

Specific syndromes such as phobias, panic attacks and obsessive-compulsive disorders (for example washing the hands continuously because of a morbid preoccupation with germs) may be part of the symptom complex.

Anxiety is generally a condition developing between the late teens and early 30s. It may be associated with substance abuse (for example caffeine, alcohol and illegal drugs). Cases occurring later in life are usually due to depressive illness.

Eighty per cent of cases resolve themselves over the course of a few weeks with reassurance and emotional support but no drug treatment. Where extreme anxiety is disrupting life, a short course of benzodiazepines (see Question 117) or of a non-addictive drug called buspirone may help. Physical symptoms such as sweating and tremor are eased by drugs which dampen nerve activity (beta-blockers) which have the advantage of being non-addictive. An anti-depressant drug will often speed recovery.

Most anxiety sufferers benefit from counselling, behaviour therapy or relaxation techniques. Those who do not respond will be referred to a psychiatrist for expert assessment of their mental state.

Recently, a brain-specific benzodiazepine receptor was discovered. This explains the effectiveness of benzodiazepines in anxiety – and has generated new theories as to the cause of anxiety and addiction. There is growing evidence that alterations in receptor function may underlie anxiety conditions such as panic attacks and alcoholism. Effective new treatments may result.

114. What can be done about phobias?

A phobia (morbid fear) is an anxiety disorder which is unreasonable, out of proportion to the cause and cannot be controlled. It is usually directed against a specific situation or object and typically, the patient will go to any length to avoid exposure to the anxiety-provoking situation. Common phobias concern spiders; snakes; mice; open spaces; crowded or small spaces; and flying. Up to 15% of men and 25% of women suffer from a simple phobia and in many cases this interferes with lifestyle and work.

Behaviour therapy using a 'systematic desensitisation' approach is a popular method of treatment where 'things', such as spiders, are involved. Pictures depicting the object of fear are shown and when anxiety occurs, relaxation techniques are used. Once the patient can cope with bigger and bigger pictures, the object itself is introduced, for example a small, dead spider in a jar. This is gradually brought closer until the patient is able to handle the jar. Eventually, a jar with a live spider will be introduced, and finally the spider will be set free.

Another technique, 'prolonged exposure', involves throwing the patient in at the deep end by exposing them to intense fear. This can be distressing, and the patient needs to be well-motivated and know exactly what is entailed. The patient has to remain in the phobic situation, without means of escape, until they acclimatise. Sessions that last at least two hours are more effective than shorter ones.

WHAT WORRIES WOMEN MOST

One in 1000 people suffers agoraphobia (fear of open spaces, going outdoors), which is twice as common in women. It often appears in the 20–40 age range and has profound social and personal implications. In many cases, depression or obsessive behaviour is present as well.

Other treatments used successfully to cure phobias are hypnotherapy, psychotherapy, creative therapy (where the patient draws or writes about the object of their fear) and group therapy.

Research is currently looking at 'visually evoked response therapy'. A patient is asked to visualise the situation they fear while moving their eyes in a certain way. Initial results are encouraging.

115. What causes post-natal depression?

There are three categories of post-natal psychiatric problems. Post-natal 'blues' occur in 50–80% of newly confined women and usually resolves within two weeks. The peak incidence is on the fifth day, with symptoms of weeping, irritability and anxiety.

True post-natal depression occurs after 10–15% of births but many cases go undetected. The majority of symptoms are short-lived but some may persist for months, even into the next pregnancy and beyond. Treatment consists of emotional support plus anti-depressant drugs if necessary (**note**: some will pass into breast milk). A significant number of cases can be prevented by administering progesterone either as injections or as suppositories, immediately after birth and for several weeks beyond. Research into the use of hormone replacement therapy using oestrogen patches looks promising.

PSYCHIATRY

The most serious of all post-natal psychiatric disorders is puerperal psychosis. This occurs in one or two out of every 1000 deliveries and is commonest after first pregnancy and Caesarean section. The sufferer may be manic or depressive with similar signs to schizophrenia. Delusions and hallucinations emerge, along with belief that the person is being persecuted. In extreme cases, the mother may even kill her baby or commit suicide.

Psychiatric assessment is essential, and a restraining order (Mental Health Act Section) is often required to admit the mother (and baby) to a specialist unit. ECT (electro-convulsive therapy) is the treatment of choice, as it gives the best chance of a rapid recovery at a time when mother-child bonding is greatly at risk. Unfortunately, there is a 20% risk of a psychotic recurrence in subsequent deliveries.

The causes of puerperal psychosis remain unclear. Personal and family histories of depression seem important, as do vulnerability factors such as lack of confidence, lack of social support and poor relationships with the baby's father. One theory is that progesterone levels are low or that progesterone receptors are faulty. Deficiency of neurotransmitters (brain chemical messengers) is possibly involved.

A recent study suggests that post-natal depression is linked with the presence of thyroid antibodies in the blood. These occur in 12% of childbearing women. Half of these will go on to develop depressive symptoms, so screening for thyroid antibodies may identify women at risk.

116. What are the symptoms of depressive illness?

The most common time for onset of depressive illness in women is 35–55 years, but it seems to appear ten years later in men. Two to three million people are affected every year, with 50% remaining undiagnosed.

A cluster of 'biological' symptoms is useful for making the diagnosis. These include sleep disturbance, especially early morning waking between 2 and 5 am; loss of appetite, with weight loss; lethargy and listlessness; weepiness; loss of sex drive; and feelings of guilt, worthlessness, or even an inclination to suicide.

Patients tend to feel worse in the morning in 'endogenous' depressive illness and improve as the day goes on. If their symptoms are 'reactive' (in response to some external factor such as bereavement, separation or unemployment) they are classically said to feel better in the morning and get worse as the day goes on. This pattern of daily variation is somewhat simplistic, however, and should not sway diagnosis too much.

Biological depressive illness is due to an imbalance of chemical transmitters in the brain. Drug treatments to correct these imbalances are very effective if administered in an adequate dose for a sufficient period of time.

Unfortunately, a MORI poll has shown that 78% of the public wrongly think that anti-depressants are addictive (they are not) and 30% believe them to be ineffective. Interestingly, 55% of those questioned reported experience of depression – 22% in themselves and 32% through a relative or friend with the condition.

Only 33% of respondents knew that biological changes in the brain were responsible for depression – although 73% felt it was a medical condition like any other illness.

117. Are sleeping tablets harmful or addictive?

The short answer has to be 'yes'. Insomnia is a common complaint which can be distressing, especially amongst the elderly. As we get older, we tend to need less sleep, partly because of inactivity and cat-napping during the day. Lying awake at night is then a normal result of going to bed too early. Getting up and doing something positive such as reading a book is the correct response, not taking a hypnotic drug.

Sleeping tablets should be used only when insomnia is severe, disabling, or causes extreme distress, for example after bereavement. Hypnotics should be used for a short time, intermittently (that is, every other night rather than every night), and certainly not taken for longer than two weeks. After this time, tolerance, dependence and withdrawal symptoms may occur.

Benzodiazepine sleeping tablets interact with brain receptors and have addictive potential. This interaction induces hypnosis but suppresses REM (rapid eye movement) sleep, which is the most refreshing. These sleeping tablets (for example diazepam, chlordiazepoxide) therefore induce a sleep which is not fulfilling. Overdose of these sleeping tablets can result in respiratory depression or irregular heartbeats (arrhythmias) and even death.

Other classes of sedative which are now proving more popular (for example antihistamines, chloral hydrate, zopiclone and anti-depressants) work elsewhere in the brain and are usually non-addictive.

The non-drug approach to insomnia involves keeping regular hours; exercising rather than sleeping during the day; relaxation therapy; and taking a warm bath before going to bed. Heavy meals, nicotine, alcohol and caffeine should all be avoided as they can all have a stimulating effect. It is important for the bedroom to be comfortable, with heat, humidity and noise kept to a minimum.

If after 15 minutes of trying, sleep still proves elusive, get out of bed, read a non-stimulating book, go for a short walk or if troubled, write down the recurrent thoughts that are keeping you awake. After half an hour go to bed again, and repeat this cycle as often as necessary. Don't just lie there and suffer hour after hour.

CANCER

Cancer is the disease women worry about most and is the second most common cause of death in the Western world. (Coronary heart disease is the number one killer.)

In the United Kingdom, a quarter of a million new victims are diagnosed every year and on average, each of us stands a one in three chance of developing cancer at some stage during our life.

Unfortunately, British women have one of the worst cancer death rates for females in Europe. Scottish women (138 deaths per 100,000) rank second only to Denmark (141 per 100,000), with women living in England and Wales coming a close third. Scottish men rank fourth (202 per 100,000) after Luxembourg, France and Belgium. Men in England and Wales are positioned in the middle of the male cancer death table. Mediterranean races, whose diet also protects them against coronary heart disease, have the lowest cancer death rates in Europe.

Over seventy per cent of new malignancies occur in patients older than 60. Surprisingly, cancer is the commonest cause of death in children between the ages of 3 and 13, with the main culprit being a form of leukaemia (acute lymphoblastic leukaemia).

'Cancer' is a term used to describe any 'corroding evil' or malignancy. It derives from the Greek word for 'crab' (*karkinos*), as ancient physicians found the irregular, jagged shapes of advanced breast cancer resembled a crab stuck to the front of the chest.

As a loose clinical term, cancer (carcinoma)

WHAT WORRIES WOMEN MOST

describes any abnormal new growth (neoplasm) associated with disordered development, invasion of adjacent tissues and the ability to spread to distant parts of the body (metastases, secondaries).

A survey in the USA suggested that up to 90% of all cancer deaths can be attributed to potentially avoidable agents. These include tobacco, alcohol, diet, sexual behaviour, occupation, pollution, and geographical features such as which country one lives in and even which side of town.

It has been estimated in the UK that tobacco is directly responsible for one-third of all cancer deaths, and doctors are now allowed to write 'smoking' as a cause of death on certificates.

118. *What are the commonest cancers?*

In Britain, lung cancer tops the list of malignant killers, accounting for 17–20% of all tumours. Over the last quarter of a century, the incidence of lung cancer has increased by 125% in men and even more in women since our consumption of cigarettes has increased. Lung cancer has now overtaken breast cancer as the most common British female malignancy.

In the UK 4200 women develop cancer of the cervix each year. The incidence is decreasing, however, due to the success of cervical screening programmes. Unfortunately, those most at risk are the ones least likely to come forward for screening. In two-thirds of cases of serious cancer of the cervix, patients have never had a smear. Worldwide, cancer of the cervix is the second most common female cancer (after breast), with around half a million

CANCER

cases occurring every year. Seventy-seven per cent of these arise in developed countries.

Cancers of the large bowel – colon and rectum – account for 11% of all deaths (male and female) in England and Wales, with skin and breast malignancies following closely at 10% each.

Skin cancers are becoming increasingly common. Malignant melanoma, a highly virulent tumour that forms secondaries very early, now accounts for 2.5% of all tumours. Exposure to the sun's radiation is the major cause.

119. Are cancers hereditary or infectious?

There is strong evidence that some cancers are linked to a transmissible agent. Carcinoma of the cervix is more common in women who have had multiple sexual partners and in women whose husbands have had multiple lovers. Women who have slept with more than six men in their life have over 14 times the risk of developing cervical cancer than those who have had no partners – or only one. In women who have had three to five sexual partners, the disease is eight times more common. This suggests a sexually transmissible agent is involved. At one time, herpes simplex virus was thought to be the culprit. Now, some of the many genital wart viruses are heavily suspected, possibly in conjunction with an as-yet-unidentified agent. Condoms do have a protective effect.

Viral particles can be identified in some malignant cells and in others, sequences of viral RNA (nuclear genetic material) have been found.

Hereditary factors play an important role. Some

WHAT WORRIES WOMEN MOST

tumours 'run' in families, for example certain rare types of cancer of the colon. Mothers, sisters and daughters of breast cancer victims are twice as likely to develop breast cancer themselves compared to women with no close relatives affected. Latest research shows the risk rises fourfold if there is also a family history of prostate cancer in their brothers, fathers or sons. An infective agent, rather than inherited genes, may of course be involved.

Exciting news is that many of these cancer genes (oncogenes) are now being identified and their DNA sequences unravelled. In future we may be able to 'switch off' tumour genes so that cancers either never develop, or regress once genes have been deactivated. A breast cancer gene has recently been tracked to a small fraction of chromosome 17. Within two years, a blood test may be available to screen for the one in 11 women who develop this disease.

120. How is cancer treated?

Not surprisingly, treatment depends on the type of cancer involved. Some are extremely susceptible to chemotherapy and others respond dramatically to radiotherapy. Some tumours are hormone-dependent, and treating with anti-oestrogens or other hormones may 'melt away' diseased tissues.

In many cases, surgery (scalpel or laser) to remove the bulk of a tumour, followed by courses of chemotherapy and/or radiotherapy, is employed. Breast removal (mastectomy) is now less common, with many surgeons favouring 'lumpectomy' followed by radiotherapy, hormonal manipulation and/or chemotherapy.

CANCER

At least 50% of cancer patients will receive radiotherapy at some stage during their treatment. Advances in imaging techniques allow pinpoint delivery of X-ray beams to selectively damage malignant cells and stop their replication. This accuracy allows less toxic doses to be given.

Radioactive needle implants are popular as they directly deliver very high doses exactly where needed.

Cancer management is among the most rapidly developing medical specialties. New, potent but less toxic chemicals are constantly being discovered, along with techniques to attach them to special antibodies. These antibodies carry the chemotherapeutic agent around the body and bind only to targeted tumour cells which the antibody recognises as 'foreign'. Normal tissue remains unaffected.

Exciting work is emerging in the field of genetics. The nuclear codes of many cancer genes are identified, isolated and sequenced almost daily. Switching these genes off, or preventing them being expressed, will soon result in many cancers being diseases of the past. Healthy gene sequences will be spliced into the DNA helix, possibly by harnessing viruses currently known to trigger tumours.

121. *What happens during a cervical smear?*

It is amazing how many women say 'Is that it?' after having their first cervical smear. It can be an embarrassing procedure but you can always request a female to take the smear for you. In many surgeries, the nurse is responsible for this test anyway.

WHAT WORRIES WOMEN MOST

At worst, having a smear taken merely feels cold. A few kind souls will remember to warm the instruments first!

A smear should not be uncomfortable at all. The women for whom it is most distressing are those who cannot relax, tense all their muscles and fight the procedure every inch of the way. This hardly ever happens. 'Virgin'-sized extra-small equipment is available if necessary.

A metal instrument (speculum) is gently inserted into the vagina to spread the walls apart, just enough to bring the cervix into view. First, the cervix is inspected for redness or suspicious lesions. Then a small wooden spatula (or a brush) is gently placed on the neck of the womb and rotated through 360 degrees. This picks up surface cells and is a totally painless procedure. The speculum is then removed.

Collected cells are 'smeared' onto a microscope slide and 'fixed' with surgical spirit until they can be stained and examined in the laboratory.

122. Should I have a cervical smear?

Every woman who has ever been sexually active should have a cervical smear. If you are over 35 and have not yet had a smear, obtaining one should be an absolute priority. It is a simple, early warning screening test which picks up 'abnormal' cells well before they become cancerous. Every year, 2000 women die from cervical cancer. Regular smears and treatment would save many of those lives.

There is some controversy over how frequently a smear should be taken. Some specialists believe once

CANCER

a year is necessary; others feel once every five years is adequate.

A sensible compromise (and the World Health Organisation ideal) is for every woman between the ages of 25 and 60 years to have a smear done every three years. Any cell abnormalities detected will result in repeat smears at more frequent intervals.

Cervical smears may only be available on the NHS every five years in your area. Check with your doctor. If you have had more than three sexual partners, your risk of developing cervical cancer is eight times that of a woman who has had fewer partners. If you have had more than six partners, your risk has increased 14-fold. In the latter case, it may be worth paying privately for an annual or three-yearly cervical smear if this screening frequency is not available on the NHS. Smokers are also at increased risk of cervical cancer.

Women who have had previous abnormal smears, or who have suffered genital warts, may be advised to have annual smears until three 'negative' results have been obtained. Thereafter the frequency may be less.

Smears are best taken mid-menstrual cycle where possible.

123. *What does an abnormal smear signify?*

Cervical smears are designed to detect early changes (dysplasia) in cells. In the majority of cases, an abnormal smear does not mean cancer, so don't panic. Your smear may be abnormal because inflammation is present, or possibly an infection such as thrush. Do not be afraid to ask your doctor exactly what is wrong, and what degree of abnormality is present.

Between normal cell appearances and microscopic changes consistent with cervical cancer, there is a continuous spectrum of cell nuclear abnormalities.

Changes described as 'mild dysplasia' frequently revert to normal. You will either be referred to the hospital for a microscopic examination of your cervix (colposcopy) or, more likely, the smear will be repeated in 3–6 months' time.

Women in whom 'moderate dysplasia' is found are usually referred for colposcopy and cervical biopsy as soon as possible, but there is no desperate urgency. These changes can still revert to normal, and often do. Frequent follow-ups are wise to detect and avoid progression to 'severe dysplasia'.

The presence of severe dysplasia makes colposcopy, biopsy and treatment urgent. Cell changes are advanced and many cells are affected. Cells have now lost their capacity for differentiation and are unlikely to revert to normal. The presence of micro-invasion, the first sign of true cancer, cannot be ruled out and progression to serious cancer may occur rapidly.

It is important that a woman should continue to use contraception between receiving notice of an abnormal smear and attending for colposcopy. Pregnancy makes treatment much more difficult. Some specialists advise coming off the pill immediately and using another form of contraception until the problem has been fully investigated. This is a precaution against hormones encouraging certain cell changes.

CANCER

124. What happens during a colposcopy?

Having a colposcopy is very similar to having a smear (see Question 121). It takes approximately 20 minutes and is usually done in a specialist hospital unit. A speculum is inserted and the cervix viewed through a microscope which remains outside your body.

The cervix is painted with dilute acetic acid (vinegar). This coagulates the protein in active areas, so abnormal cells and wart virus infection shows up white. Sometimes the cervix is painted with an iodine solution; abnormal areas fail to stain brown.

The microscope allows the most abnormal areas to be identified and biopsied. If an area is obviously very abnormal, treatment may be started there and then on the basis of your smear report. In most cases, treatment is postponed until the result of the biopsy is through.

Treatment aims to kill abnormal cells in a localised manner. Abnormal cells are destroyed by burning with a laser or, more usually, with diathermy (electrical heat). Sometimes a cone biopsy is performed, where a cone-shaped piece of the cervix is cut away. This has the advantage of supplying tissue for a thorough microscopic examination but, if too much is taken, an 'incompetent' cervix may cause problems during future pregnancies. A local anaesthetic is used during these procedures.

The only discomfort felt tends to be 'cramping', which has been described as similar to very bad period pains.

CELLULITE

125. What is cellulite and how can it be minimised?

Cellulite gives the skin a mottled, dimpled appearance reminiscent of an orange skin. It is due to the bulging of over-loaded, subcutaneous fat storage compartments. Connective tissues are compressed and blood and lymph vessels draining the area become narrowed. Fat cells are increasingly undernourished as excess fluid and waste products (toxins) build up. This results in further compression of tissues and a vicious circle evolves.

Over several years, fat cells harden giving established cellulite its characteristic waxy, lumpy feel. Oestrogen may be involved as men do not seem to suffer – though their fat compartments are also larger.

The best remedy for cellulite is to follow a low-fat (especially low saturated fat), low salt diet with high levels of natural source minerals and vitamins. These are obtained from fresh, raw or lightly cooked fruit and vegetables. Carbohydrate intake should increase to compensate for lowering dietary fats.

A minimum total fluid intake of three litres per day is advised – preferably in the form of mineral water. Additives, highly processed foods, tea, coffee and alcohol are best avoided. Smoking is detrimental to elastic tissues in the skin and will encourage sagging, wrinkles and cellulite.

Regular exercise tones flabby muscles and stimulates the circulation. Many women have found help

CELLULITE

from regular massage, especially with aromatherapy oils. Dry skin brushing with a bristly vegetable brush is said to stimulate lymph flow.

As a last resort, cosmetic surgery is available. During liposuction, fat cells are dissolved and removed via a syringe. Lipo-endolase therapy, newly developed in France, uses a tiny endoscope and a laser to eradicate excess adipose fat. Both techniques involve cutting the skin and may leave scars.

INDEX OF MEDICAL QUESTIONS

Abnormal Smear	185
Abortion	43, 44
Acne	138–140
Ageing Skin	129–137
Aids	25, 27
Alcohol	159–162
Alcohol Dependency	161
Anal Sex	22
Anorexia Nervosa	155
Anxiety	171
Bone Density Screening	115
Breast Cancer	118–123
Breast Implants	125, 126
Breast Lumps	118, 120
Breast Milk	77
Breast Pain	122
Bulimia	155
Calories	149
Cancer	179–187
Cellulite	188
Cervical Smear	183, 184, 185
Cholesterol	142
Collagen Injections	130
Colposcopy	187
Combined pill	33, 36
Contraception	32–45
Contraceptive Injection	41
Cosmetic Breast Surgery	124–128
Cystitis	79–81

What Worries Women Most

Depressive Illness	176
Diaphragm	39
Emergency Contraception	37, 38
Endometriosis	96
Episiotomy	76
Excess Body Hair	135
Exercise	157
Face Lift	133
Fat	151
Fibroids	94
Frigidity	19
G-Spot	20
Genital Thrush	85
Healthy Diet	141–147
HIV	25, 27
Hormone Replacement Therapy (HRT)	104
HRT Patch	108
Hysterectomy	93–101
Infertility	59–66
Mammogram	121
Masturbation	23
Mediterranean Diet	146
Menopause	102–117
Menstrual Cycle	46
Metabolism	151
Mini-Pill	35, 37
Miscarriage	71
Morning-After Pill	37

INDEX

Oral Sex	21
Orgasm	16, 17
Osteoporosis	113
Ovaries	99
Pelvic Inflammatory Disease	96
Periods	46–54
Pheromones	29
Phobias	173
Post-Menopausal Bleeding	109
Post-Natal Depression	174
Pre-Conception Preparation	68
Pre-Menstrual Syndrome (PMS)	55–58
Pregnancy	67–78
Prolapse	95
Psychiatry	168–178
Safer Sex	28
Sex	15–31
Sex Drive	18
Sexually Transmitted Diseases	24
Sleeping Tablets	177
Slimming	148–158
Slimming Pills	153
Smoking	163–167
Sperm	23
Spots	138
Sterilisation	42
Stress Incontinence	82–84
Stress Levels	169
Stretch Marks	134
Symptoms of Stress	168
Thrush	85–87

WHAT WORRIES WOMEN MOST

Toxic Shock Syndrome	53
Tretinoin	132
Vaginal Discharge	88–92
Very Low Calorie Diet	154
Virgin	15
Vitamins	156
Wrinkles	130

OTHER BOOKS IN THE PICCADILLY POINTERS SERIES

PROBLEM PERIODS – Causes, Symptoms, and Relief
by Dr Caroline Shreeve

STAYING TOGETHER – The Secrets of a Successful Relationship
by Belinda Hollyer

STRONG ENOUGH FOR TWO – Women Taking the Strain in a Relationship
by Liz Roberts

FINDING THE LOVE OF YOUR LIFE – Using Dating Agencies and Ads
by Linda Sonntag

ADVENTURE UNLIMITED – Living and Working Abroad
by Suzanne Askham

SINGLE AGAIN – Living Alone and Liking It
by Anita Naik

ARE YOU READY YET? – Preparing for a New Relationship
by John Gordon

INSIDE MEN'S MINDS – Young Men Talk
by Nick Fisher